THE OVERTHINKER'S RESCUE PLAN

7 Days To Clear Your Mind,
Make Better Decisions, and Reclaim Your Focus

Grant Merrill

Copyright © RWCM, LLC

The Overthinking Overthinker's Rescue Plan,
Copyright © 2025 RWCM, LLC.

Paperback ISBN: 979-8-9991913-1-1

All rights reserved. No part of this book may be reproduced or used in any manner without written permission of the copyright owner except for the use of quotations in a book review. Thank you for your support of the author's rights.

The scanning, uploading, and distribution of this book without permission is a theft of the author's intellectual property.

First paperback edition June 2025

Published by RWCM, LLC, All rights reserved.

Contents

Introduction: Why You're Here (and What You'll Leave With) 1

Chapter 1: Awareness – Identifying Overthinking Patterns 4

Chapter 2: Clarity – Distinguishing Productive vs. Unproductive Thoughts 19

Chapter 3: Mindfulness – Staying Present in the Moment 33

Chapter 4: Decision-Making – Building Confidence in Choices 47

Chapter 5: Boundaries – Managing Information and Commitments 61

Chapter 6: Self-Compassion – Embracing Imperfection 74

Chapter 7: Integration – Creating Sustainable Habits 86

Bonus Section: Your Reset Toolkit & Ongoing Support 97

Suggested Reading List and Maintaining Progress 101

From the Author, Grant Merrill 109

About the Author 111

Introduction: Why You're Here (and What You'll Leave With)

Let's be honest: you are here because you're a dynamic, driven individual who consistently gets things done. In fact, you juggle multiple responsibilities, navigate complex problems, and manage the countless details of both your professional and personal life with apparent ease. Yet, despite this outward calm and success, there is an undercurrent that never quite stops churning. Your mind refuses to switch off, even when it should.

You find yourself replaying conversations long after they have finished, questioning whether you said the right thing. Decisions haunt you long past the point where all facts have been gathered and assessed. And then, in those quiet moments meant for rest, you lie awake pondering: Did I overlook something crucial? Should I be doing more?

Sound familiar? If so, take a breath. You're not broken; you're simply overthinking. This book exists to tell you that you're not just understood—you're in the exact right place to transform that relentless mental energy into something powerful and liberating.

This isn't another book filled with theoretical discourse or academic jargon. You don't need more theory; you need practical solutions—a reset that seamlessly fits into your real life, one that respects your limited time while supporting your significant ambitions. This book is crafted specifically for curious minds like yours—individuals who are perpetually "on," always engaged in mental multitasking. You may feel stretched between ambition and exhaustion, yearning for clarity but trapped in cycles of second-guessing. It's time to cut through the noise with purpose.

I've designed a focused, 7-day plan aimed at delivering real results quickly. With short chapters, actionable tools, and immediate results, this journey promises transformation without overwhelming your already packed schedule.

Over the next seven days, you will be introduced to foundational skills essential for mastering your mind:

The journey begins with awareness. On day one, you'll learn to spot the recurring patterns in your thinking. Recognizing these habits is the first step toward redirecting your thoughts productively.

Next, we delve into clarity. Day two will teach you how to filter thoughts to prioritize those that genuinely serve your goals and well-being. This skill is crucial for decluttering your mind.

Mindfulness comes on day three, equipping you to focus deeply in any given moment. Discover the peace found in presence, significantly reducing stress.

On the fourth day, decision-making is our focus. You'll learn to make choices with confidence, freeing yourself from the endless cycles of doubt and hesitation.

Day five introduces boundaries. Protecting your time and energy becomes second nature, enabling you to guard against burnout while honoring your own needs and priorities.

Self-compassion takes center stage on day six. We are often our toughest critics; you'll learn to replace negative self-talk with understanding and patience, fostering a healthier relationship with yourself.

Finally, on day seven, we integrate these skills, turning them into sustainable habits. The journey concludes with techniques to ensure these changes endure, enhancing your mental landscape for the long term.

The format is straightforward. Each day's focus includes worksheets, reflection prompts, and concise actions tailored to fit into even the tightest of schedules. Whether you can spare five minutes or thirty daily, you'll experience meaningful progress and a tangible shift in how you engage with your thoughts and emotions.

The aim here isn't to reinvent yourself; rather, it's about uncovering and nurturing the calm, clear, capable version of yourself that exists beneath the constant stream of mental chatter. By committing to this process for just one week, you open the door to profound shifts. You'll make decisions faster, conserve energy by dialing down mental noise, and cultivate a sense of focus, grounding, and control like never before.

So, if you're ready to embark on this transformation, let's reset together—one decisive day at a time.

Chapter 1: Awareness – Identifying Overthinking Patterns

Sarah sat at her desk, staring once again at the email she had just sent. The cursor blinked mockingly as she reread every word for the third time, searching for errors that weren't there. Minutes stretched into hours, yet she couldn't press "send" on the follow-up message to her client. Her mind spun through all the possible mistakes she might have made, each one more unlikely than the last, but the doubt gnawed relentlessly at her confidence. Meanwhile, her to-do list grew longer, meetings loomed closer, and her fatigue deepened.

This experience is familiar to many professionals who find themselves caught in endless cycles of overthinking—an automatic mental trap that drains energy and stalls progress. Such patterns often go unnoticed, disguised as thoroughness or responsibility, leaving busy individuals struggling to move forward despite their efforts. Understanding how these thought habits form and learning to recognize their signals creates a crucial first step toward gaining control. This chapter will guide you in developing a clear awareness of your unique overthinking tendencies by identifying common patterns, distinguishing your personal triggers, and adopting practical approaches to redirect unproductive loops of thought.

Understanding the Importance of Awareness and Recognizing Overthinking

Habits, including overthinking, are formed through repetition. In workplaces where stress, high expectations, and constant decision-making are common, behaviors become ingrained as a way of coping. Neural pathways strengthen each time a person responds to uncertainty with the same thought process, building automatic responses over time. This means overthinking isn't a character flaw but a learned pattern, driven by practice rather than personality. Recognizing this is essential. When people see overthinking as a habit, they realize it's possible to replace it—just as any other automatic habit can be unlearned and replaced with something healthier.

Awareness serves as the light that reveals these mental habits. In busy professional lives, it is easy for overthinking to go unnoticed under the justification of responsibility or diligence. Without awareness, people unconsciously reinforce these patterns, mistaking rumination or analysis paralysis for effective problem solving. Genuine change only becomes possible when someone sees their thinking not as inherent, but as something developed and maintained through consistent responses to stress and pressure.

Overthinking manifests in several recognizable patterns in professional environments. A manager who sends a project update and then rereads the sent email multiple times is not practicing diligence, but demonstrating analysis paralysis—an endless review stemming from fear of making a mistake. An executive spends restless nights mentally rehearsing every detail of their presentation, believing it will prepare them, but instead sinking into catastrophic thinking about what could go wrong. A team lead finalizes a decision in a meeting, only to spend the next hour double-checking outcomes in their mind, replaying conversations, and doubting choices, trapped in rumination. These examples illustrate how overthinking actively drains time, energy, and focus, often disguised as thoroughness.

Overthinking Pattern Recognition Exercise

Pattern: Analysis Paralysis

Purpose: Analysis paralysis involves freezing in the face of decisions, endlessly gathering data or reviewing tiny details in search of perfect certainty.

Real-world example: A project manager receives a draft report from a direct report. Instead of providing timely feedback, the manager spends hours reviewing every sentence for errors, then hesitates before sending comments, double-checking even routine points.

Indicators:

Physical: Jaw tension, fidgeting at the desk, eye fatigue from rereading screens.

Mental: Racing thoughts about potential outcomes, indecision over minor details.

Emotional: Frustration, self-doubt, feeling stuck.

Common misconceptions: Believing "thorough" always means "better," or that more analysis guarantees the best outcome.

Pattern: Catastrophizing

Purpose: Catastrophizing occurs when the mind jumps to the worst possible outcome, inflating minor setbacks into impending disasters.

Real-world example: After a tense team meeting, a department head worries that a colleague's brief disagreement signals deep dissatisfaction, imagining consequences like losing the team's trust or being reported to upper management.

Indicators:

Physical: Racing heart, shallow breathing, trouble settling thoughts.

Mental: Persistent focus on what could go wrong, exaggerating risks.

Emotional: Anxiety, nervousness, dread.

Common misconceptions: Assuming preparing for every negative outcome means being responsible, or that worrying prevents bad results.

Pattern: Rumination

Purpose: Rumination is repeated replaying of past events with focus on flaws, regrets, or perceived failures, long after the event has passed.

Real-world example: After delivering feedback during annual reviews, a leader reruns the conversations all week, criticizing their tone or word choice, asking themselves if they were misunderstood or too harsh.

Indicators:

Physical: Sleeplessness, headaches, ongoing fatigue.

Mental: Looping thoughts about the same event, inability to let go.

Emotional: Regret, guilt, irritability.

Common misconceptions: Thinking self-reflection is always positive, ignoring when it becomes unproductive dwelling.

Busy professionals experience these patterns in response to demanding roles. Overthinking frequently masquerades as preparation or responsibility, but a closer look reveals tolls on well-being: loss of sleep, mental fatigue, increased anxiety, and reduced ability to remain present at home and work. Empaths—those especially sensitive to the emotions of others—are more prone to such patterns, as they absorb tension from their environments, further complicating their emotional lives.

As patterns become visible, people may notice that certain scenarios—crucial presentations, performance evaluations, difficult conversations—tend to activate these habits. By simply paying close attention to mental activity around key situations, readers start identifying where their patterns most frequently emerge, preparing to pinpoint triggers in the next stage of change.

The Three-Column Overthinking Log

This exercise promotes direct awareness by encouraging self-observation rather than self-judgment.

Situation	Thought pattern observed	Impact on work/wellbeing
Reviewing a sent email	Analysis paralysis—rechecking every word for mistakes	Delayed response to new emails, increased tension
Prepping for quarterly review	Catastrophizing—imagined all possible failure scenarios	Sleep disruption, irritability toward team

Capturing these entries brings overthinking from the background into conscious focus. Each time this is practiced, it strengthens the foundation for future change, setting the stage for deep exploration of triggers that drive these habits.

Spotting Your Triggers and Applying Awareness at Work

Recognizing External and Internal Triggers During the Workday

Busy professionals often encounter a blend of external and internal factors that spark overthinking. External triggers include looming deadlines, an avalanche of emails, ongoing workplace disagreements, and ever-shifting project requirements. For example, a manager might notice growing anxiety as a critical deadline approaches, leading to extended hours spent double-checking every detail of a report. Similarly, a team member tasked with responding to a high-volume inbox could find themselves stuck in a cycle of revising drafts of a single email, overanalyzing word choices for fear of misinterpretation. Virtual meetings bring their own set of external triggers; the ping of an incoming call just before a scheduled presentation can initiate a worry spiral: Will the technology fail? Did I prepare enough slides?

Internal triggers, such as perfectionism and imposter syndrome, also fuel overthinking. A new department head with high personal standards may obsess over refining a project plan, fearing that any flaw will diminish their reputation. This "project planning paralysis" can slow decision-making and sap productivity when the need for flawless execution overshadows realistic progress. Imposter feelings—persistent worries about being "found out" as incompetent—can surface during team feedback sessions, fueling doubts after even mildly critical input. The professional then replays every comment in their mind, wondering if their competence is in question. These internal triggers frequently result in excessive self-criticism, emotional exhaustion, and a sense of falling behind despite continual effort.

To move from vague unease to actionable self-awareness, tracking exercises can offer valuable daily insights. Recognizing the constraints on professionals' time, the following system requires only brief, intentional moments during naturally occurring work breaks.

A Workplace Trigger-Tracking Template

Trigger Identification Method

Begin by observing specific moments when stress, indecision, or a racing mind sets in. Use environmental cues—such as the start of a meeting, the reception of a new email, or feedback from a supervisor—as prompts to note internal reactions. Look not only for obvious stressors but also subtler signals like hesitation before speaking up or repeatedly rewriting a simple client update.

Implementation Steps

Identify a trigger in real time. Pause for one or two breaths when noticing a stress surge, tight shoulders, or repeated negative thoughts.

Record the context and the nature of the overthinking: was it deadline pressure, perfectionism, imposter worries?

Use a notepad, sticky notes, or a digital note app for quick, private recording—no elaborate tracking system required.

Log the specifics: when, where, what happened, what you noticed in your response.

Expected Insights

By reviewing these notes at the end of the day or week, patterns begin to emerge. Many discover that certain meetings, emails from specific colleagues, or particular types of tasks elicit disproportionate rumination. Small but recurring cues—like dreading virtual video calls or hesitating to submit routine reports—gain clarity as repeating triggers.

Application in Daily Work Routine

Consistent use of this tracking method during commute times, coffee breaks, or between meetings quickly builds a personal checklist of workplace "hot spots." Over time, this raw trigger data forms the foundation for deeper analysis and the development of strategic responses.

Exercises to Build Trigger Awareness

The Quick Trigger Scan (2 Minutes)

Timing: Mid-morning, ideally after the first major task or meeting.

Action Steps: Stop, close your laptop (or look away from your phone), and mentally scan for moments since your arrival when your thoughts spiraled: pre-meeting jitters, hesitating over a difficult email, or rehashing a colleague's feedback.

Professional Context: This approach works equally well in remote or office settings, before a coffee refill or a restroom break.

Progress Marker: If you can quickly name one or two triggers without hesitation, your awareness is growing.

The Workplace Pattern Log (5 Minutes)

Timing: Immediately following a recurring event—such as a weekly team check-in or project handoff.

Action Steps: Jot down the trigger, your internal response, and how it influenced your actions (did you delay submitting work, overprepare, or ask for unnecessary reassurance?).

Professional Context: This method is adaptable for all roles and is particularly useful for leaders after giving presentations or for executives after analyzing financial reports.

Progress Marker: Repeated entries of the same trigger signal a pattern ripe for further exploration.

The End-of-Day Reflection (3 Minutes)

Timing: Before leaving work (or during your commute if you are using public transit, or while waiting for a rideshare).

Action Steps: Briefly review your day's entries or recall key stressful moments. Note which triggers had the greatest impact and which strategies helped—or did not help.

Professional Context: This reflection is effective for sales professionals recalling client calls, IT analysts reviewing incident tickets, or HR team members following mediation sessions.

Progress Marker: Awareness of shifts in trigger frequency or intensity over the course of a week.

Seamless Integration Into the Workday

Incorporating these quick scans does not require changes to your schedule. Use coffee breaks, the brief window before a virtual meeting begins, or the few minutes between tasks for check-ins. Cues to notice include an increased heart rate before giving a presentation, procrastination at the start of a solo project, or tightness in the chest during difficult team collaborations. Repeated use of these strategies equips professionals with the raw observations necessary for more detailed pattern recognition later on.

Labeling Thought Loops and Building Sustainable Daily Awareness

Defining and Naming Thought Patterns

Thought patterns are the habitual ways your mind processes similar situations. They are predictable, recurring themes or loops that capture your attention and often shape your behavior. For busy professionals, these thought cycles intensify under stress, making it essential to recognize and label them quickly for effective management.

Step-by-Step Guide to Identifying Personal Thought Loops

Begin by pausing the next time you notice racing thoughts interfering with your focus. Pinpoint the topic or event that is sparking these thoughts. Write down every distinct idea that repeats or nags at you throughout the day. After doing this for several days, review your notes to identify the patterns that appear consistently.

These patterns reveal your brain's default concerns, worries, and self-talk cues.

Creating Personalized Thought Tags

With your recurring thought loops identified, assign each one a simple, memorable label: a "thought tag." This tag transforms abstract worries into concrete, nameable items, making it easier to spot them when they arise. Keep each tag short and descriptive so you can recall it on the fly and instantly ground yourself.

Common Thought Pattern Examples

Presentation Perfectionism Loop: "I must have every detail right before showing my work. Any flaw means failure."

Decision Doubt Spiral: "What if I make the wrong call? Should I double-check this with someone else?"

Client Feedback Loop: "Did my client's short reply mean they're unhappy? Should I follow up or let it go?"

Imposter Syndrome Echo: "People will realize I'm not as competent as they think."

Urgency Catastrophe Cycle: "If I don't handle this now, everything will fall apart."

Thought Pattern Documentation Template

Pattern Name	Description	Triggers (People/Events/Time)	Intensity (1-10)	Frequency (per day)

Fill in your top three recurring thought patterns, noting the context surrounding their appearance. Mark their intensity and frequency. This tracking turns intangible worries into actionable data.

Daily Awareness Anchoring

Boost your awareness by implementing consistent, structured check-ins. Select three specific times that align with your work rhythm: before your first major task, midday, and just before finishing. These check-ins prevent ruminative thoughts from dominating.

Check-In Structure

Morning Start (before your first task)

What am I thinking about as I begin work?

Are any familiar thought tags present already?

Midday Reset (right after lunch or at the halfway point)

Have any thought patterns persisted?

What impact are they having on my productivity or mood?

End-of-Day Wrap (as you prepare to leave or log off)

Which patterns dominated today?

Did I catch any early and redirect my attention?

Physical Anchoring Methods

Anchor your commitment to these check-ins by placing physical reminders where you will see them: sticky notes on your monitor with your three thought tags, a small reference card in your wallet, or reminder alarms on your phone labeled with your tags (e.g.,

"Check: Perfectionism?"). These tangible cues train your brain to pause, observe, and label thoughts regularly.

The 5-Minute Mind Dump

At each check-in, set a timer for five minutes. Grab a notepad or a digital note. Write freely about anything looping through your mind, tagging recurring patterns as you spot them. Format:

Time of day and check-in

Stream-of-consciousness thought notes

Tag each thought pattern as it comes up (e.g., "[Decision Doubt Spiral]")

Stop at five minutes. This brief, unfiltered release recalibrates your attention and gives structure to scattered thinking.

Real-World Professional Scenarios

A sales executive routinely launches into the "presentation perfectionism loop" every time a new pitch is scheduled, delaying completion while obsessing over minor tweaks. Labeling this pattern, he places a sticky note on his laptop: "Perfection is Not Required—Send It." At each check-in, he tracks whether the urge to over-polish arose before submitting.

A manager recognizes the "decision doubt spiral" when assigning tasks to her team. During lunch, she uses her phone to note every decision she hesitated over that morning, asking, "Did the spiral slow me down?" Phone alarms prompt her to tag those thoughts and redirect her focus before her next meeting.

A consultant receives terse client feedback, instantly triggering the "client feedback loop." At her end-of-day check-in, a quick journal prompt asks, "Did I read too far into that email?" Tracking this helps her disengage emotionally and reset for the next day.

Tracking Progress

Use concrete metrics:

Number of unique thought patterns tagged by end of week

How many times each pattern was caught and labeled daily

Percentage of times patterns were detected early versus after the fact

Days where productivity was measurably higher after catching and anchoring patterns

Set automated reminders, color-coded sticky notes, and index cards with tag definitions on your desk for fast reference. Use journal prompts: "Which pattern showed up most? Did naming it help me move forward?".

Consistent practice in naming and tracking thought patterns, paired with daily checkpoints and visible reminders, builds clarity and control for busy professionals. Each named pattern loses its power to ambush your attention and begins to reveal opportunities for productive change.

Summary and Reflections

Now that we understand how to recognize overthinking patterns, identify their triggers, and apply daily strategies for awareness, we are equipped to take meaningful steps toward regaining control over our thoughts. By consistently observing and labeling these mental habits, busy professionals can break free from unproductive cycles that drain energy and focus. This growing self-awareness lays the foundation for intentional change, enabling us to replace automatic overthinking with clearer, more effective thinking. Moving forward, this chapter's tools prepare us to face challenges with greater calm and confidence, fostering healthier mental habits that support success both at work and beyond.

Chapter 2: Clarity – Distinguishing Productive vs. Unproductive Thoughts

Clarity of thought is often elusive in the fast-paced world of busy professionals. Imagine sitting at your desk, confronted by a flood of competing thoughts—some urging you to act, while others drag you into endless worry. One moment, your mind jumps to a nagging concern about an upcoming presentation; the next, it spirals into doubts about your capabilities and potential failure. The line between helpful reflection and counterproductive rumination blurs, leaving you mentally exhausted and unsure of where to focus your energy. These experiences are common, yet few stop to recognize which thoughts actually deserve their attention and which merely consume time without producing results.

This constant mental noise can lead to missed opportunities and unnecessary stress, especially when decisions must be made quickly or when managing complex team dynamics. Without a clear way to distinguish productive thinking from unproductive cycles, professionals risk being overwhelmed by distractions that hinder progress. Learning how to identify and manage these different types of thoughts is essential for maintaining focus, reducing stress, and maximizing effectiveness. This chapter presents approaches to help you recognize which mental patterns signal actionable insight and which are simply noise, offering practical methods to develop clarity amid the demands of a busy workday.

Defining Mental Clarity and Identifying Thought Quality

Mental clarity, for busy professionals, means deliberately managing thoughts to create space for rapid decisions and reduced stress. It is not about silencing the mind but about sorting, prioritizing, and acting only on thoughts that truly support goals. In business settings where team conflicts, looming deadlines, or challenging presentations often collide, mental clarity becomes the edge that keeps professionals focused, resourceful, and efficient throughout the day.

Consider the moment when a team conflict erupts. One stream of thought might immediately spiral into frustration: "This always happens in my team. Why can't people just cooperate? This is exhausting." Another thought emerges: "I see two team members disagreeing about roles. What can I clarify to reduce this tension right now?" The first sequence leads to ruminative worry, while the second pinpoints a specific role in resolving the conflict. Mental clarity is the ability to recognize the difference—choosing actionable, forward-focused thoughts over those that trap you in stress and indecision.

Staying clearheaded is practical, not abstract. In preparing for an important presentation, unfiltered anxiety might produce the thought: "I'm going to mess up this presentation, and everyone will lose confidence in me." Instead, productive thought management allows for the thought: "I need to practice the opening twice and review key data points. If a question throws me, I will pause, repeat the question, and give myself time." The difference shows up in actual performance—productive thought selection leads to rehearsal and strategic planning, which cut prep time and boost delivery.

At the core of this chapter are two frameworks to help professionals distinguish thoughts that fuel action from those that amplify overwhelm.

The Productive vs. Unproductive Thought Test offers a simple diagnostic. Each thought can be evaluated with three questions. First, does the thought prompt a meaningful action? Next, does it offer an opportunity for growth or learning? Finally, does it energize you to act, or does it loop in circles? When a project deadline looms, a professional may think: "I will never finish all of this in time." This thought neither triggers action nor teaches anything new—classify it as unproductive. The revised thought, "What are the three tasks I must complete today to stay on track?" creates an action list and sharpens focus—meeting both action and growth criteria. The immediate impact is that energy shifts from anxiety to action, shortening task initiation times.

The Signal vs. Noise Framework takes this further, dividing workplace thoughts into two clear categories. Signal refers to actionable insights that lead to solution steps; noise marks those patterns that keep the problem alive without drawing any closer to resolution. Applying this framework to handling emails, a professional may notice: "My inbox is overwhelming; I'll never get through it." This is noise—circular thinking with no solution. The signal is: "I'll set a timer for 20 minutes, scan for urgent client emails, and archive the rest." Action follows, and the number of unresolved emails shrinks in real time.

Three workplace examples anchor these frameworks in the realities busy professionals face:

Scenario One: Meeting Preparation

During a meeting run-through, you catch yourself thinking: "If I say something wrong, I'll embarrass myself." You apply the Productive vs. Unproductive Thought Test:

Action potential: None, it just fuels worry.

Learning: No new insight.

Classification: Unproductive.

By contrast, "Prepare two key points and a question to ask the group," ticks action and learning—productive. Applying Signal vs. Noise, "What are the biggest potential objections?" is signal, guiding preparation. "What if nobody likes my idea?" is noise.

Scenario Two: Project Planning

When tackling a new initiative, you catch: "There's too much to do; it's hopeless." Productive/Unproductive test: no action, no growth—unproductive. Swapping for "Start by mapping milestones, then delegate one piece today" checks both boxes—productive. Signal is recognizing, "Identifying early hurdles now will save double the time later." Noise sounds like, "What if I forget something important?"—cycling with no output.

Scenario Three: Team Feedback

Post-feedback session, you think: "They probably think I'm too critical." No action, just rumination—unproductive and noise. Alternatively, "After feedback, ask team for their perspective next time," prompts action and reflection—productive and signal.

Every day is filled with thousands of thoughts. Most are distractions or repetitions that slow response, foster fatigue, and block result-oriented thinking. Professionals who systematically distinguish signal from noise—and productive thoughts from unproductive ones—train their mental "filters" to support rapid, confident action.

Preparing for the Clarity Scan practice ahead, begin by recognizing thought patterns as either energizing "signals" that prompt solutions or as wearying "noise" that trap you in worry. The division is not theoretical; it is a learned, daily skill with measurable outcomes: faster decisions, sharper focus, and more effective communication with your team.

Filtering Thoughts and Navigating the Gray Areas

The daily Clarity Scan exercise is a focused check-in that helps busy professionals instantly sort their thoughts, giving immediate clarity on what moves you forward (signal) and what distracts you (noise). The core purpose is to filter thoughts for action and release, supporting sharper decisions and calmer focus throughout the day. This practice directly applies the Signal vs. Noise Framework: instead of wrestling with every thought, you learn to filter, act, or let go in the moment—a skill that builds clarity and momentum.

The method starts with pausing for a quick internal scan, especially when your mind feels crowded or your energy drops. Core steps take no longer than three minutes and can be used multiple times daily.

Clarity Scan: Step-by-step Implementation

Thought Capture Moment (30 seconds): Pause and notice what thought is occupying your mind. Write it down or state it clearly in your mind.

Outcome Identification (30 seconds): Ask, "What is the desired result if I address this thought?" Name the outcome in concrete terms.

Action Possibility Assessment (60 seconds): Decide if there is a real, immediate action you can take to influence the outcome. Explicitly state the action or acknowledge if it is outside your control.

Decision Point (release or proceed, 30-60 seconds): If actionable, proceed and take the next step; if not, deliberately let the thought go. Tell yourself, "I am releasing this thought for now."

Consistently following these steps helps transform overloaded thinking into productive action or peaceful release. Use this scan during short breaks, before meetings, or when switching tasks.

Expected Outcomes

Faster decisions and less time stuck in indecision

Noticeably lower stress levels

Greater energy and focus for important work

Improved follow-through because only actionable thoughts get attention

Professionals who use the scan report more satisfaction with their workdays, as unproductive mental clutter decreases.

Common Pitfalls

Skipping the outcome identification step and acting without direction

Looping on the same unproductive thought without releasing it

Forgetting to track whether a thought is within your control

Remind yourself that indecision is a cue to return to the scan steps and use physical signals as prompts.

Clarity Scan in Action: Real-World Examples

Work-Related Scenario: Meeting Preparation

Initial thought pattern: "I'm worried my update at the meeting will sound unprepared."

Filtering process:

Capture: "Worried about sounding unprepared in update."

Identify outcome: "Want to deliver a clear, confident update."

Action assessment: "Can I act now? Yes, review key points and confirm updates."

Decision: Proceed—spend ten minutes outlining points.

Resulting action: Review and rehearse. Tension in shoulders eases, and focus improves.

Personal Decision Scenario: Contemplating Career Change

Initial thought pattern: "Maybe I should switch industries, but what if it's a huge mistake?"

Filtering process:

Capture: "Thinking about industry change, worried about mistakes."

Identify outcome: "Want job fulfillment, less regret."

Action assessment: "Immediate action? No, research is needed first—set time to investigate top options."

Decision: Proceed—schedule 30 minutes for market research tonight.

Resulting action: Plan research, release worry for now. Notice a drop in scattered thinking and improved mood.

Relationship Scenario: Team Conflict

Initial thought pattern: "I think my teammate dislikes my approach—should I confront this today?"

Filtering process:

Capture: "Team conflict concern."

Identify outcome: "Want open, collaborative relationship."

Action assessment: "Is there something to do now?" Yes, clarify feedback and invite discussion during team check-in."

Decision: Proceed—frame an invitation for conversation.

Resulting action: Send a brief message to open dialogue, feel energy shifting from anxious to proactive.

Handling Gray-Area Thoughts

Set timeframes: If a thought lacks a clear action, calendar five minutes tomorrow to reassess—decide then, not now.

Transform vague worries: Change "Will this project fail?" to "What is one thing I can do today to move this project closer to success?"

Journaling prompts: Use quick prompts like "Is this within my control?" or "What is the smallest next step?"

Workplace Applications

Email processing: Run a Clarity Scan before responding—does this email require action, information, or polite archiving?

Meeting participation: Scan your objectives at meeting start and focus only on thoughts linked to those goals.

Project planning: Apply the scan to task lists; release low-impact items.

Decision-making moments: Pause, scan outcomes, act only on high-impact thoughts.

Recognizing Physical Cues

Common markers of unproductive thought patterns include tightness in shoulders or jaw, drained energy at midday, and trouble refocusing after distractions. These cues signal a need for a Clarity Scan break.

Metrics for Progress

Track time saved per decision, reduced stress at day's end, and percentage of actionable versus released thoughts each week. Noticing increased completed actions and better emotional well-being means your filtering skill is building strength, preparing you for the next level of mental clarity.

Building the Clarity Habit: Training Skills and Leveraging Tools

Busy professionals often think of mental clarity as a passive state, unlocked only during rare moments of calm. In reality, clarity is a skill that can be practiced and strengthened much like a muscle. The key is to move from simply observing your thoughts to engaging in directed mental training. This practice, called Clarity Muscle Training, builds on daily clarity scans and thought filtering by introducing repeatable exercises designed for work-life demands.

Clarity Muscle Training centers on three focused exercises: Pattern Recognition, Micro-Reset Protocol, and the Thought Filter Exercise. Together, these practices form a sequence that builds mental strength, cuts through cognitive clutter, and transforms workplace stress into actionable insights.

Clarity Muscle Training

Pattern Recognition Exercise

Definition: Pattern Recognition asks you to clearly notice recurring thought loops and automatic emotional responses—without judging or reacting to them.

Implementation Steps:

Set a timer for 3 minutes once daily, ideally before your first meeting.

Sit comfortably and write down the first thoughts that surface about your workday.

Scan those thoughts for repeated themes, such as "I always dread team calls" or "I worry projects will run late."

Mark each repeated pattern with an asterisk.

Expected Results: By regularly tagging recurring patterns, you increase your awareness of triggers, build objectivity, and reduce anxiety in future similar situations. This exercise lays the foundation for conscious decisions rather than reactive habits.

Troubleshooting Tips: If you notice self-judgment, remind yourself that the goal is simple identification. If themes seem vague, ask a peer if they notice similar patterns and compare notes.

Time required: 3 minutes

Optimal time: Early morning

Materials: Notebook or digital note app

Success metrics: Number of distinct thought patterns logged each week

Micro-Reset Protocol

Definition: Micro-Resets create rapid, energizing breaks that clear mental fog between tasks or meetings.

Implementation Steps:

Stand and perform three slow shoulder rolls, followed by ten deep breaths (about 60 seconds).

Close your eyes and name the next immediate task aloud to yourself.

Conclude by taking one conscious step away from your current workspace, then physically return.

Expected Results: Improved energy, enhanced focus, and fewer mental carry-overs from previous meetings. With repeated practice, transitions between tasks become smoother and less mentally taxing.

Troubleshooting Tips: If the reset feels rushed, use a reminder to slow your movements. If your mind drifts, focus on a single inhale and exhale.

Time required: 1-2 minutes

Optimal time: Between meetings or after completing a task

Materials: Quiet space

Success metrics: Number of resets completed per day; reported level of energy or focus right after the reset

Thought Filter Exercise

Definition: This worksheet-based tool helps you evaluate automatic thoughts and choose those that serve your professional goals.

Implementation Steps:

At the end of the workday, jot down any stressful or persistent thoughts.

For each thought, use the 5-question checklist to assess validity and relevance (see below).

Record answers and action steps directly on the worksheet.

Expected Results: More filtered, intentional thoughts; a reduction in circular mental chatter; and clearer next actions.

Troubleshooting Tips: If you feel stuck, read your answers aloud to check for realism. If worksheets multiply worries, limit it to two main thoughts per day.

Time required: 5 minutes

Optimal time: End of day

Materials: Printed or digital worksheet

Success metrics: Number of thoughts processed and filtered; actions identified

Using the Clarity Calendar

Log brief notes about recurring thought themes, triggers, and moments when you applied an exercise. Color-code for patterns (e.g., red for anxiety, green for successful resets). Review entries each Friday for trends. If you spot a cluster of high-stress entries related to certain meetings or people, use that data to refine your reset or filtering practices the following week.

5 Questions to Filter Any Thought

For each workplace scenario, such as negotiating with a difficult colleague:

Is this thought true?

(Did the colleague actually disagree with me, or am I assuming?)

Is this thought helpful right now?

(Does worrying move the project forward?)

What evidence supports this thought?

What evidence refutes it?

Is there a constructive action to take?

Use these questions in situations like urgent project delays or unclear feedback. The checklist targets unproductive thoughts and drives practical responses.

Case Studies

Case 1: Alex, a mid-level manager at a tech firm, noticed growing dread before weekly standups. Pattern recognition revealed that this anxiety peaked after status updates. After three weeks of using the micro-reset and thought filter, Alex reduced meeting stress, participated more, and led a major project shift decisively.

Case 2: Priya, a marketing director, logged repeated thoughts of "falling behind." By tracking these in her Clarity Calendar and adjusting with guided resets, her productive thinking hours increased, while self-reported stress dropped by 40% over a month.

Tracking Progress

Monitor the number of interrupted thought loops daily, compare time blocks spent in focused work versus worry, list concrete actions generated by each filter review, and measure changes in stress through daily check-ins.

Each element of Clarity Muscle Training builds precision into mental habits, creating a robust, trainable clarity skill set.

Bringing It All Together

Now that we understand how to distinguish productive thoughts from unproductive rumination using practical frameworks and the Clarity Scan, busy professionals can take deliberate control of their mental focus. By consistently applying these repeatable processes, individuals will reduce wasted energy on worries that do not serve their goals and instead channel their attention toward actionable insights. This intentional filtering strengthens mental clarity as a skill, enabling faster decisions, lower stress, and greater effectiveness in both daily tasks and complex challenges. Moving forward, practicing these techniques will build lasting habits of clear thinking, ensuring sustained productivity and resilience amid workplace demands.

Chapter 3: Mindfulness – Staying Present in the Moment

In the fast-paced world of professional life, moments of distraction and mental overload are all too common. Picture a busy executive juggling emails, meetings, and looming deadlines, only to find their mind wandering to unfinished tasks or incoming notifications. This constant mental drifting not only hampers focus but also fuels a cycle of overthinking that erodes productivity and heightens stress.

Such experiences reveal a widespread challenge: maintaining clear, purposeful attention amid the relentless demands of modern work. Understanding how the mind can become fragmented by distractions is essential for anyone seeking to perform at their best without succumbing to overwhelm. This chapter delves into practical mindfulness strategies designed specifically for busy professionals. It emphasizes accessible techniques that help recognize distractions, manage thoughts, and return to present tasks with renewed clarity—without requiring lengthy meditation or retreat-style practices. The goal is to equip you with straightforward tools to sharpen focus, reduce cognitive fatigue, and enhance your effectiveness in the workplace.

Understanding Mindfulness and Its Impact on Overthinking

Mindfulness is often misunderstood as a mystical practice reserved for yoga studios or long meditation retreats, but for the modern professional, it is better defined as the skill of directing your attention with intention. In the context of a demanding workplace, mindfulness means noticing when your focus drifts from the task at hand, recognizing distractions, and actively redirecting your attention to your priorities. This approach turns mindfulness into a cognitive tool, no different from project management software or data dashboards—something to train and deploy for sharper performance. Successful professionals who practice mindfulness skillfully maintain clarity during high-stakes client calls, juggle shifting priorities across multiple tabs and projects, and respond to unexpected requests without losing composure or productivity.

Clearing Common Myths

Misconceptions prevent many from exploring mindfulness as a business asset. One myth suggests that mindfulness requires emptying your mind or achieving total calm. Modern professionals rarely have time to sit cross-legged in silence, and fortunately, mindfulness doesn't demand that. Instead, it involves catching yourself when your focus slips to an incoming Slack message or when pre-meeting nerves ramp up, then steering your attention back to the requirements of the current project.

A second myth equates mindfulness with relaxation or disengagement. In reality, mindfulness sharpens engagement. You perform a quick scan of your inbox for urgent messages, identify unnecessary worries about last week's sales figures, and realign your priorities without spiraling into anxiety. Attention control, not relaxation, drives this process.

A third misconception suggests that mindfulness is only for those with plenty of extra time. Even during hectic days packed with meetings and deliverables, integrating mindful moments—such as pausing briefly before dialing into a video conference—can reset your focus and prevent mental fatigue. These brief interventions, rather than hour-long sessions, support professionals in maintaining optimal performance.

Boosting Productivity Through Attention Mastery

Workplace productivity rises and falls based on the quality of attention management. When you notice your mind darting to an unfinished slide deck during a one-on-one with your manager and redirect your focus to the conversation, you strengthen the neural patterns associated with attention control. This produces concrete results: faster task completion, reduced error rates, and easier transitions between competing demands.

Mindfulness also reduces the toll of decision fatigue. Constant interruptions and switching between tasks create a cognitive drain. By training yourself to notice when you drift—such as toggling between calendar invites and project updates—and pulling your focus back to a single deliverable, you conserve mental resources and make clearer choices. Enhanced communication clarity follows: when you listen closely in meetings instead of mentally rehearsing your response, you ask sharper questions and resolve issues faster.

Overthinking, Stress, and the Science Behind Mindfulness

Overthinking—or cognitive rumination—manifests at work as repetitive worry about what went wrong or what's next, driving up stress hormones like cortisol. Research from leading business schools and neuroscientific studies demonstrates that professionals who consciously monitor and direct their attention experience lower baseline cortisol levels. In practice, less circulating cortisol translates to improved impulse control, better problem-solving, and an increased ability to prioritize under pressure.

For example, when a sudden project scope change hits your inbox, the initial spike in worry can lead to scattered thinking, missed deadlines, or excessive email re-checking. Mindfulness interrupts this feedback loop. By training yourself to notice the onset of runaway thoughts and returning to the specifics of the new requirements, you stabilize your attention and respond systematically rather than reactively.

Exercise: The Awareness Audit

Purpose: The Awareness Audit helps pinpoint your current habits regarding attention—you discover whether you tend to get swept up in browser tab chaos or regularly lose track of discussions in meetings.

Method: Choose a typical workday. Set brief reminders at random intervals—this can be a calendar alert or a sticky note—and, at each cue, log what you are focusing on at that moment. Note any distractions, task switches, or automatic routines (such as skimming social feeds or jumping between drafts).

Application: With this snapshot, patterns become clear: perhaps your focus fades after receiving Slack pings, or your thoughts drift during status updates. Use these insights to make small changes: mute non-essential notifications during critical work, summarize key meeting points immediately after they finish, or take a slow, mindful sip of coffee before tackling your next priority.

Hectic work environments present daily challenges—mounting emails, meeting anxiety, and shifting expectations. Tools like the 5-4-3-2-1 Reset or Box Breathing can address these issues, empowering professionals to act with clarity. Understanding mindfulness as attention management—not a mystical escape—lays the groundwork for leveraging these targeted techniques in practical, high-impact ways.

Quick Mindfulness Techniques and Their Application at Work

Tension gathers unnoticed as professionals juggle urgent emails, pop-up meetings, and shifting priorities. Overthinking can hijack the mind in these work moments, making it challenging to focus or act decisively. Practical micro-mindfulness techniques offer a way to regain clarity without stepping away or needing special equipment. Essential to their success is the ability to act in seconds, making them especially useful in busy work environments.

5-4-3-2-1 Reset

This method uses sensory cues to shift your mind from racing thoughts to the present. Brain science shows that engaging multiple senses redirects attention from stress pathways to the rational, calmer parts of the brain. This technique proves useful for professionals before high-pressure meetings or presentations, when anxiety spikes or focus wavers.

How it works:

Sit upright at your desk and plant your feet flat on the ground.

Name five things you can see (e.g., your screen, a mug, a pen).

Name four things you can feel (e.g., the chair's support, the watch on your wrist).

Name three things you hear (e.g., the keyboard, a distant conversation).

Name two things you can smell (e.g., coffee, the office air).

Name one thing you can taste (e.g., mint, tea).

This process grounds your mind using external stimuli and interrupts rumination almost immediately.

Time required: 40–60 seconds

Physical and mental response: Slowed heart rate, eased muscle tension, increased clarity.

Workplace example: Before a client call, where last-minute nerves threaten performance.

Success indicators: Calmer breathing, steadier voice, renewed attention.

Troubleshooting: If a sense is unavailable, skip and continue; if distractions occur, restart from the last completed step.

Box Breathing

Box Breathing, also called square breathing, helps regulate the nervous system. Research illustrates that measured, intentional breaths signal safety to the brain, reducing stress chemicals. Employees facing multiple deadlines or shifting tasks can use this technique to stay composed and alert.

Implementation:

Inhale for 4 seconds.

Hold the breath for 4 seconds.

Exhale for 4 seconds.

Hold again for 4 seconds.

Repeat this cycle for four rounds.

Time required: 64 seconds for four cycles.

Physical and mental response: Slower pulse, clear-headedness, increased control.

Office scenario: While switching between urgent projects, you feel overwhelmed and scattered.

Success markers: Shoulders drop, thinking becomes more organized, and the urge to rush lessens.

Troubleshooting: If you lose count, glance at a clock or tap your fingers to stay on beat; if you yawn, it's a sign that your body is relaxing.

The Mindful Sip

Simple acts, like sipping a drink, can interrupt autopilot states and support mental resets. Research shows that pairing physical activity (like drinking) with mindful attention temporarily "pauses" automatic stress responses, making it easier to regain present focus. Afternoon energy slumps or difficult conversations often benefit from this small but powerful approach.

Step-by-step:

Hold your cup and feel its surface.

Smell the drink's aroma for 3 seconds.

Take a slow sip.

Notice the temperature, texture, and taste.

Let your exhale last as long as possible after the sip.

Repeat twice.

Time required: 30–40 seconds

Physical and mental cues: Relaxed jaw, softened gaze, and less frantic energy.

Application: When facing a difficult feedback session, use this technique while reviewing notes or just before entering the meeting room.

Success indicators: Slower speech, easier eye contact, and steadier hands.

Troubleshooting: If you get interrupted, mentally recall the taste or feeling for a moment to anchor yourself back.

Exercise 1: Workplace Reset

Stand or sit upright and perform the 5-4-3-2-1 Reset exactly as shown above.

Duration: 60 seconds

Notice your breathing deepening and your hands unclenching.

Check: Has your inner monologue slowed? Are your thoughts more orderly?

Suggestion: Use this after returning from lunch or when you return to your desk after an interruption.

Exercise 2: Mindful Task Transition

Before you click into a new task, pause.

Take 2 rounds of Box Breathing (32 seconds).

Stand and stretch your arms over your head for 10 seconds.

Notice: Has your urge to "rush in" decreased? Is your focus clearer?

Success: Your mind feels reset, and anxiety about "what's next" quiets.

Action: Jot down a single intention for the next task on a sticky note.

When a trigger appears—like an urgent request, a difficult conversation, or an overloaded inbox—identify which cue fits your experience. Choose the matching technique (sensory grounding for nervousness, breath work for overwhelm, mindful sipping for recalibration). Apply the method immediately and observe the response. If stress lingers, repeat once or combine with brief stretching. Short, consistent practice after common workplace triggers helps these techniques become natural, automatic responses over time, supporting your balance and resilience even on the busiest days.

Making Mindfulness Stick: Habits, Handling Distraction, and Extra Support

Connecting mindful moments to habits already built into your day transforms mindfulness from an extra task into an integrated routine. Habit pairing attaches a brief practice to an existing action. For example, pause and take a slow breath before opening your inbox, let your hands relax on your laptop with every password entry, or ground your feet before entering a meeting room. These pairings become automatic reminders, seamlessly blending mindfulness into tasks that professionals already perform without adding more to their workload.

Anchor moments offer a simple way to establish a foundation for consistent practice. An anchor moment is a reliable point in your daily routine that cues a brief mindful pause. Strong anchors include the first sip of morning coffee, putting on a headset to join a virtual meeting, logging off at the end of the day, or starting your commute home. The anchor must be consistent and personally meaningful, making it a natural "reset point" regardless of how busy the day feels. For remote workers, entering a dedicated workspace or opening a laptop can become the anchor, while office professionals may use swiping a keycard or greeting colleagues. Choose an anchor that resonates with your daily rhythm, not just one that is convenient.

A personalized approach avoids overwhelm and increases sustainability. A "Mindfulness Menu" is a toolkit of three practices tailored to your work style and common stressors. For example, someone in frequent meetings might choose a grounding breath, a mood check, and a tension release as their three tools. Someone with a creative job may select a sensory scan, a two-minute mindful note, and a pausing technique before brainstorming sessions. Having this menu ready prevents decision fatigue, so you know exactly what to use when you need it most.

The Notice → Name → Return method helps busy professionals break the cycle of distraction and refocus with clarity.

Notice: Become aware of where your mind is right now. Recognize distractions without judgment.

Example: While reading emails, realize that your attention drifts to an unfinished task.

Challenge: The tendency to ignore or push away distractions.

Solution: Gently acknowledge the distraction as normal.

Indicator of Success: You spot distractions sooner.

A simple 3-Minute Reset practice can re-center your mindset amid a hectic schedule.

3-Minute Reset Interactive Workbook

Purpose: Briefly refresh focus and ease tension during the workday, even in high-demand roles.

Implementation:

Name: Label what you notice—"worried," "planning," "tired."

Example: Name the feeling of tension before an important call: "anxious."

Challenge: Difficulty labeling or fearing judgment.

Solution: Use broad, neutral words. There is no need for accuracy, only awareness.

Indicator of Success: Emotional responses feel less intense.

Return: Bring your focus back to your chosen anchor or task.

Example: After naming "anxious," direct your attention back to the next action on your calendar.

Challenge: Your attention keeps wavering.

Solution: Repeat the process without frustration.

Indicator of Success: Shorter transitions back to focus.

Day	Time	Sensory Prompt	Awareness Noticed	Reflection
		What do you hear, see, or feel?	What body sensation or thought caught your awareness?	What shifted in your productivity or mood afterwards?

Begin with three deep breaths.

Scan for sensory details (the sounds of colleagues, the hum of electronics, and clothing against your skin).

Expected Benefits: Sharper attention, fewer energy slumps, and a better workplace mood.

Troubleshooting: If you are distracted, start with a single sensory check (such as hearing) and expand gradually.

Progress Markers:

More regular use of the reset (track it for one week).

Noticing fewer moments of overwhelm before midday.

Increased ease in returning to work tasks.

Mindfulness Hack Checklist for Work

Take a conscious breath before responding to difficult messages.

Ground yourself before presentations (feel your feet against the floor).

Notice three details in a meeting (color, sound, gesture).

Stand up slowly and notice your posture at transitions.

Set a calendar reminder for micro-breaks.

Jot down a quick note on what you discovered.

Use reflection prompts: "What changed in my stress level after the reset?" "Was it harder or easier to focus?"

Customizable Cue Card Template

Trigger	Mindful Response
Phone rings	Relax shoulders
Video call connects	3 slow breaths
Feel tension rising	Name the emotion
End of work session	Stretch and scan body

Personal Reset Recording Guidelines

Record a brief reminder in your own voice to guide you through the 3-Minute Reset.

Use simple cues: "Pause, breathe, notice one sound, return."

Dealing with inconsistency means focusing on system cues and tracking. Use metaphors like "closing mental browser tabs" whenever you take a mindful breath, helping to reboot attention and clear lingering distractions. If practice drops off, gently return to your anchor moment and restart with just one small pairing rather than trying to catch up all at once. With repetition, these small resets become a professional's natural workflow, preparing a strong foundation for future advanced applications.

Bringing It All Together

Now that we understand mindfulness as a practical tool for managing attention amid the demands of a busy workday, professionals can confidently integrate these accessible strategies to reduce overthinking and enhance focus. By embracing brief, intentional moments of awareness—whether through sensory grounding, controlled breathing, or mindful pauses—we build resilience against stress and improve productivity without disrupting our workflow. With consistent practice and personalized cues, mindfulness becomes an automatic ally that sharpens decision-making, sustains mental clarity, and supports sustained performance in any professional environment. This foundation prepares us to face future challenges with calm, control, and greater effectiveness.

Play it at scheduled points for a consistent routine.

Chapter 4: Decision-Making – Building Confidence in Choices

Every day, busy professionals face an overwhelming number of choices—from deciding what to eat for breakfast to managing complex work priorities and responding to countless emails. This constant stream of decisions slowly drains mental energy, making even simple choices feel exhausting and fraught with doubt. Often, the hesitation isn't about lacking information but a fear of making the wrong move, which leads to wasted time, increased stress, and stalled progress.

This chapter examines how indecision quietly saps confidence and productivity. It highlights the hidden toll that endless weighing of options takes on the mind, explaining why striving for perfection can backfire. Through understanding these challenges, readers will be guided toward strategies that restore decisiveness and encourage action, helping them overcome paralysis and build trust in their choices.

Understanding Decision Fatigue and the 'Good Enough' Shift

Every day, the average adult makes around 35,000 decisions, from choosing breakfast to replying to emails and scheduling meetings. This sheer volume of choices leads to a mental drain known as decision fatigue. Consider a busy professional approaching lunchtime, faced with dozens of food options, each requiring small judgments. Multiply that by every tab open, each email awaiting action, and every request for their attention. By mid-afternoon, even straightforward decisions—like responding to a colleague's query or prioritizing which file to finish first—become difficult as mental reserves deplete over time. Constant, rapid-fire decision-making drains cognitive resources, leaving professionals sluggish and prone to errors.

The tangible costs of decision fatigue manifest in wasted time, rising stress, and reduced productivity. For instance, an executive may spend ten minutes dithering over whether to accept a meeting, only to lose focus on the next task. A team leader might re-read the same email thread repeatedly, unable to decide on a response, effectively wasting valuable time. Small choices, when repeated throughout the day, accumulate and slow down overall progress. This inefficiency often results in missed deadlines, forgotten details, and an increase in minor mistakes. Research highlights how decision fatigue can lead to avoidance behaviors, such as procrastination or defaulting to easy, less optimal options.

Contributing to this spiral is the physiological impact: stress hormones increase, motivation drops, and emotional regulation weakens. Over time, professionals experiencing decision fatigue may notice that they snap at colleagues, postpone tough calls, or feel overwhelmed by seemingly simple choices. The accumulation of unresolved decisions creates mental clutter, resulting in burnout and a sense of helplessness. According to leading experts, when demands in personal and professional life overlap, the lines blur, amplifying stress and making it more challenging to recover energy.

At the root, the main psychological barrier is not a lack of skill or information, but the fear of making the wrong choice. This anxiety leads to decisional paralysis. Many professionals know which option is reasonable yet hesitate, apprehensive about negative consequences or regret. For example, a manager with all the facts about delegating a project might freeze from the fear that the team will disapprove or that results will falter. Similarly, a project lead may have clear priorities but still lose time agonizing, imagining worst-case scenarios if the chosen action backfires. Understanding that decision-making blocks often stem from emotional resistance rather than knowledge gaps is crucial.

A practical way to break out of paralysis is to reframe decisions as experiments instead of permanent, all-or-nothing choices. This mindset shift reduces anxiety by allowing professionals to see decisions as opportunities to gather feedback rather than definitive measures of ability. When experimenting, the cost of a suboptimal outcome is learning, not failure. For instance, a supervisor unsure about switching to a shorter meeting format can commit to trying it for two weeks, evaluate feedback, and refine the structure based on results. An employee uncertain about whether to delegate a routine report can do so once, observing results and making adjustments if needed. Framing decisions this way removes the weight of needing every choice to be perfect and increases the willingness to act.

Another practical application is the "Good Enough" rule. This rule suggests that decisions do not need to be flawless; 80% confidence is often sufficient to proceed. Practically, reaching 80% confidence means you have most key facts, have weighed the main risks, and believe the option will work under typical conditions. There may be some uncertainty, but the potential gains outweigh possible drawbacks. Chasing 100% certainty leads to diminishing returns as more time is spent combing through minor variables rather than acting. Perfectionism can actually reduce effectiveness, as delayed decisions freeze progress and increase backlogs.

Workplace examples support this approach. A product manager quickly selecting a "good enough" design for a feature based on available user data, rather than waiting for all possible testing, will likely refine the product faster as real-world feedback rolls in. An HR director who approves a new onboarding schedule after conducting a partial pilot, rather than waiting for exhaustive consensus, accelerates improvements and reduces bottlenecks. In both cases, a willingness to accept "good enough," rather than perfect, results in faster progress and better morale.

Mindset shifts—seeing decisions as experiments and aiming for "good enough" outcomes—empower professionals to reclaim their time. This approach redirects mental energy from endless deliberation to learning and real-world execution. With a clear understanding of these psychological and practical strategies, professionals can now consider frameworks and tools to implement efficient, confident decision-making. These strategies pave the way for tangible, sustainable productivity gains within fast-paced, modern workplaces.

Applying Fast Decision-Making Tools and Building Trust in Your Choices

The 3-2-1 Method offers a streamlined structure for making timely choices. Its core principle is containment: limit both the number of options under consideration and the time spent evaluating them. This approach curbs analysis paralysis by directing focus and activating decisive action.

To implement the 3-2-1 Method, start by identifying three viable options. Narrow these down to your top two. Set a visible five-minute timer to compare the final two, then select one winner. For example, when choosing between candidates for a key project management role, review three top resumes, interview two, and extend the offer to one. For a personal purchase, such as a home, shortlist three properties, schedule viewings of the top two, and submit an offer on one by the end of the day.

Common pitfalls include overcomplicating initial options (trying to include more than three) and failing to enforce the timebox. Success indicators are reduced regret, a completed decision within your set window, and clear next steps taken immediately after deciding.

Exercise: Activate the 3-2-1 Method

Objective: Make one concrete decision in 10 minutes.

Materials: Pen, paper, timer.

Time Limit: 10 minutes.

Success Metric: One decision made, with the next action written.

Next Step: Act on your selected choice before reviewing the process.

The Cost-of-Delay Check helps assign real consequences to indecision. Its central principle is conscious quantification: make the daily price of waiting visible. To calculate, list the tangible results lost for each day of delay: lost revenue, missed opportunities, and wasted time. For a career example, delaying a job offer decision by three days could cost you $600 per day in potential earnings and prevent onboarding, pushing back project timelines. With personal health, delaying a physiotherapy appointment adds another day of discomfort, possibly compounding the problem and increasing long-term costs.

To use this framework, write the decision to be made at the top of a page. Underneath, list time, money, and missed opportunity costs for every day undecided. Total these for the most realistic impact assessment.

Common pitfalls include underestimating opportunity costs and failing to act on the insights generated. Success means a rapid decision, reduced anxiety over abstract "what-ifs," and a clear sense of the value created by timely action.

Exercise: Complete the Cost-of-Delay Check

Objective: Quantify and minimize costs of indecision.

Materials: Spreadsheet or notebook.

Time Limit: 7 minutes.

Success Metric: Written cost breakdown with total daily loss.

Next Step: Decide within the next 24 hours and execute the associated action.

The 10-10-10 Rule strengthens perspective by evaluating possible outcomes over three time horizons: 10 minutes, 10 months, and 10 years. Its core idea is temporal distancing—separating short-term emotion from long-term importance.

In practice, identify the decision and write answers to these prompts:

How will I feel about this in 10 minutes?

How will I feel about this in 10 months?

How will I feel about this in 10 years?

A senior manager considering whether to accept a demanding promotion may feel overwhelmed now, uncertain in 10 months, but see it as a career-defining pivot in a decade. For everyday decisions, such as joining a new gym, the initial inconvenience may disappear, but improved health and confidence persist for years.

Common pitfalls involve answering superficially and failing to identify genuine emotions versus passing frustrations. Success appears as reduced reactivity and increased alignment with enduring priorities.

Exercise: Apply the 10-10-10 Rule

Objective: Assess decisions with clarity across time.

Materials: Journal and pen.

Time Limit: 8 minutes.

Success Metric: Three written responses detailing perspectives at each time point.

Next Step: Choose the option with a positive future impact and implement your choice.

After any decision, reinforce confidence with a Decision Anchor Sheet. This one-page template roots decisions in core values, not fleeting emotions, and guides forward steps. Compose:

Decision statement (be specific)

Three supporting values (e.g., integrity, growth, impact)

Three key factors considered (data, stakeholder needs, timing)

Two next actions

Success comes from seeing a clear connection between values and decisions, reducing second-guessing.

Exercise: Create Your Decision Anchor Sheet

Objective: Ground your choice in values-based reasoning.

Materials: Printed template, pen.

Time Limit: 10 minutes.

Success Metric: Complete sheet with clear action steps.

Next Step: Display your sheet in your workspace and check off actions as completed.

Apply the decide and redirect technique to turn mental churn into momentum. Replace "But what if this fails?" with "Now I will move forward by…" For a product launch, instead of revisiting launch readiness, say, "Now I will inform the team and begin rollout." For personal decisions, change "I'm not sure I made the right call" to "Now I will follow through for 90 days, then review results."

With these tools, you gain not only a process for making decisions but also new language for carrying them forward. Individual frameworks like these, once mastered, set the foundation for collaborative decision-making in teams, scaling personal confidence into shared momentum.

Collaborative Decisions and Overcoming Persistent Indecision

Teams achieve progress when they have clear protocols for decision-making and systems for overcoming indecision. Professionals who apply well-defined strategies reclaim their mental energy and consistently keep projects moving forward. Streamlined group dynamics and actionable self-management tools prevent wasted time and lower stress for everyone involved.

Team Decision-Making Protocols

The Time-Box Method

Teams use this method to limit endless discussions. Cap group input at 15 minutes to prevent over-analysis.

Implementation Steps:

State the problem and specify the 15-minute limit.

Allow each member one minute for input.

Summarize points and facilitate a quick poll or vote.

Announce the decision and move forward.

Real-World Example:

In a project kickoff, the team faces two design options. The lead says, "We have 15 minutes for feedback, one minute each. Keep comments focused on our primary client need. At 10:30, we'll decide." Timers are set, input is brief, and the design is finalized within the set constraints.

The DRI (Directly Responsible Individual) Approach

Assign a single decision-maker for every task or domain. This streamlines accountability, clarifies ownership, and accelerates outcomes.

Implementation Steps:

Designate the DRI at the outset of each initiative.

Announce their role in meetings and documentation.

Provide the DRI with the authority to make the final call after collecting team input.

Real-World Example:

During resource allocation, the product manager is named the DRI for timeline changes. Team members submit data and recommendations. After considering the input, the manager sets the new deadline and communicates it company-wide.

The 2-5-1 Framework

Force decisions through structure: limit choices to two clear options, set a five-minute total discussion timer, and require one outcome.

Implementation Steps:

The leader narrows options to two.

The team debates pros and cons for five minutes.

Once time is up, the group votes, or the DRI makes the call.

Real-World Example:

A sales team is split between targeting two key accounts. The manager presents: "We have five minutes to weigh both. At the end, we'll pick one to pursue this quarter." Action is taken without prolonged debate.

The "No Without Guilt" Framework

Professionals maintain focus by declining nonessential tasks firmly and empathetically.

Scripts for Declining Requests

"Thanks for thinking of me, but I can't take this on right now due to existing priorities."

"I appreciate the opportunity. At the moment, my workload won't allow me to give this the attention it deserves."

"I'm going to pass on this request to stay focused on my current commitments."

"I don't have the capacity for new projects, but I can recommend someone else who might help."

Email Templates for Postponing Commitments

"Thank you for reaching out. My schedule is full this week; can we revisit this next Tuesday?"

"I'd like to give this proper attention, but timing is tight. Could we circle back mid-month?"

"Currently, I am unable to commit. Can we schedule a review call in two weeks?"

Conversation Models for Renegotiating Deadlines

"Given my workload and project priorities, is it possible to adjust the deadline by one week to ensure quality?"

"I want to deliver my best work. What flexibility do we have in the timeline to accommodate shifting priorities?"

Breaking Through Persistent Indecision

Overthinking Diagnostic Tool

Physical Signs of Decision Paralysis:

Tension or tightness in the shoulders and neck

Repeatedly checking the same documents

Inability to sit still

Delaying responses to emails or calls

Headaches or fatigue during decision periods

Mental Indicators:

Circular thoughts about possible outcomes

Frequent "what if" scenarios without conclusion

Difficulty prioritizing clear next steps

Rapid Intervention Techniques:

Say "I've made my decision" aloud.

Close the mental browser tab: write your choice and stop reviewing reasons.

Commit to the first-best solution.

Confirm with a peer or mentor in two minutes.

Do a "gut-check" and trust your initial instinct.

Use a timer: give yourself five minutes to finish.

Identify the smallest actionable next step and do it immediately.

Professional Context Examples:

Allocate a marketing budget: use the 2-5-1 framework. Lead a project: name a DRI. Decide between vendors: time-box to 15 minutes. Handle overthinking with rapid intervention to prevent delays.

Permission to Act Framework

Coin-Flip Scenarios:

Two equally strong project solutions with no clear winner.

Choosing between two partners for a pilot.

Settling a tiebreaker during team votes.

"Good Enough" Thresholds:

Meets the client's main need.

Delivers within budget.

Satisfies 80% of requirements.

Achievable within the next two business days.

Approved by at least two stakeholders.

Two-Minute Decision Drill:

State your two best options. List pros and cons in writing. Take a breath and decide. Commit to act on it immediately.

Done is Better Than Perfect Assessment Tool

Qualifying Questions:

Does this solve the immediate problem?

Will delays seriously impact results?

Is further refinement likely to bring major benefits?

Have I received sign-off from key stakeholders?

Does this version meet core requirements?

Action Triggers:

Mark the task as complete in your workflow.

Notify the team of your final decision.

Deliver the outcome to the intended recipient.

Commitment Statement:

"I will move forward with this solution and focus my energy on the next priorities."

Using these protocols and tools turns decision-making from an energy drain into a manageable, empowering process.

Final Thoughts

Having explored the causes and consequences of decision fatigue, as well as practical mindsets and tools to overcome it, busy professionals are now equipped to reclaim their mental energy and act with greater confidence and speed. By embracing the good-enough mindset, using rapid decision frameworks, and applying clear protocols both individually and in teams, readers can break free from indecision and perfectionism that hinder progress. Now that these strategies are understood, professionals can move forward decisively, reducing stress and boosting productivity while fostering a culture of effective, value-driven choices that sustain momentum in demanding work environments.

Chapter 5: Boundaries – Managing Information and Commitments

Every day, professionals find their workdays bleeding into their personal time. An unexpected email lands during dinner, a phone call interrupts the evening, or a meeting creeps into what should have been a moment of rest. These moments are often dismissed as unavoidable; yet, they slowly chip away at focus, energy, and well-being. The constant influx of information and demands can leave even the most dedicated individuals feeling drained and overwhelmed.

This chapter examines how setting clear boundaries is essential for managing the flow of information and commitments in both professional and personal spheres. By establishing limits around time, communication, and emotional engagement, busy professionals can protect their focus, sustain productivity, and maintain their mental health amid the pressures of modern work life. Practical strategies are presented to help reclaim control over one's schedule and interactions, enabling sustained performance without sacrificing personal well-being.

Understanding Boundaries and Their Impact

Boundaries allow busy professionals to define where work ends and personal needs begin. In a demanding workplace, boundaries serve as protectors of time, attention, and emotional energy. Think of boundaries as invisible lines drawn around your workday, conversations, and thoughts. Without clear boundaries, urgent emails invade your evenings, team crises interrupt your lunch, and stress seeps into every corner of your routine. Professionals need boundaries to deliver their best work without running on empty.

Boundaries are not barriers or signs of weakness; they help individuals safeguard their focus and well-being. For instance, if you decline that "quick meeting" that always overruns into your lunchtime, you are not rejecting your team—you are setting a limit that protects your health and keeps your mind sharp. If you inform your manager that you turn off notifications after six o'clock, you create space for rest and show respect for your off-hours. These are everyday examples of boundaries in action.

Professional boundaries carry significant weight because the workplace often blurs personal and professional needs. Employees share goals, deadlines, and challenges, as well as stress and emotional struggles. If a colleague is overwhelmed, you may take on their tasks out of guilt or loyalty. While this might help in the short term, you may soon find your own priorities slipping. You check emails at dinner, cover others' shifts, and agree to more than you can handle. Over time, this leads to exhaustion, resentment, and mistakes.

The costs of weak boundaries manifest in several ways. Constant interruptions—from messages, meetings, and colleagues—make it difficult to complete complex tasks. Research highlights that people waste up to 28% of their workweek managing interruptions, with distractions lowering productivity and increasing errors. When professionals set no limits, quality suffers. You miss details, lose motivation, and fail to meet deadlines. Team morale also declines, as overloaded employees may become impatient or withdraw from collaboration.

Mental well-being also depends on boundaries. If you cannot disconnect from work calls or emails, stress accumulates, leading to burnout. Prolonged exposure to work stress erodes confidence and makes individuals vulnerable to anxiety and depression. For support professionals, the risks multiply; absorbing clients' or colleagues' stress can lead to vicarious trauma or compassion fatigue. Such experiences distort your worldview and drain your emotional reserves. Over time, you become less helpful to others and more likely to leave your job.

Without clear boundaries, work invades personal life. Projects spill past deadlines, leaving no time for exercise or family. Quick tasks at night turn into extended work sessions. As you neglect your needs, your health suffers, relationships weaken, and job satisfaction evaporates. This makes it difficult to advance in your career or earn recognition. Ambitious professionals who try to "do it all" without boundaries eventually struggle to keep up. Their efforts become spread thin, achievements are overlooked, and promotions slip out of reach.

Effective boundaries look different depending on the context. They fall into three main types: time, information, and emotional.

Time Boundaries

Time boundaries protect your schedule. For example, you might block out a daily hour for focused work or insist that you do not attend meetings during lunch. If a client expects a reply outside of business hours, you can inform them that you respond within business times. Calendar blocks, auto-responses, and downtime reminders all help create time boundaries.

Information Boundaries

These boundaries determine what information you share or receive. You have the right to keep personal matters private at work. For instance, you might limit work discussions during family events or refuse to gossip about colleagues. With digital tools, strong information boundaries can involve setting rules about who has access to your contact information or how you handle sensitive files. When work communication is constant, clear agreements about when to reply and what to share can help curb overload.

Emotional Boundaries

Emotional boundaries protect your feelings and mental space. Supporting a grieving coworker is compassionate, but you can say, "I'm sorry, I can't talk about this right now" if you feel drained. When a colleague vents every day and it weighs on you, a healthy limit might involve guiding them to professional support. Emotional boundaries prevent you from being swept up in the problems of others or taking criticism personally. If you find yourself waking up at night worrying about work, your emotional boundaries need attention.

Workplace technology often pressures individuals to relax these limits. Smartphones, chat platforms, and video calls enable instant access but erode the boundaries that once protected focused work and rest. Colleagues in different time zones, urgent notifications, and blurred home-office lines require professionals to become boundary-setters. With practice, stating and upholding boundaries becomes a strategic asset, not just for self-care but for delivering high-impact results and setting an example for colleagues.

Implementing Boundaries at Work and Home: Practical Strategies

Every day, busy professionals face a flood of emails, meeting requests, and shifting expectations from leaders, colleagues, and clients. Maintaining productivity and well-being depends on establishing strong boundaries to separate meaningful work from shallow demands. Two exercises, focused on digital boundaries and the art of saying "no," offer concrete ways to protect both time and attention—key elements for thriving in demanding professional environments.

Digital Boundary Implementation

Email remains a top source of information overload for professionals. Shifting away from treating the inbox as a task list reclaims mental energy and enables deeper focus. By dedicating three specific times for checking email—9:15 a.m. (after an initial deep work block), 1:15 p.m. (post-lunch), and 4:30 p.m. (as the workday winds down)—inboxes are checked consistently but not compulsively. Between these times, email apps are closed, and phone notifications are silenced.

The one-minute rule provides immediate clarity: if an email takes less than sixty seconds to answer, do it during a batch-check session; if not, add the task to a focused work list, not the inbox. For example, if a remote project manager receives a request for a meeting link, it can be sent and scheduled on the spot. However, a contract review inquiry, which requires thirty minutes, should be added to the next day's deep work calendar block.

Calendar blocking is essential for carving out "deep work zones." A concrete example is to add a hold event labeled "Client Deliverable:

No Calls/Emails—Protected Focus" from 10:00 a.m. to 12:30 p.m. each morning. Set the calendar status to "Busy—Working on High-Priority Project" with the following status message: "Current block reserved for focused work. Please email; I will respond during my next scheduled check at 1:15 p.m." This transparent language helps team members set their own expectations, reinforcing information and time boundaries.

Measurable outcomes for this new system include tracking the number of work interruptions due to email (expect at least a 50% reduction), the number of tasks moved from email to formal to-do lists, and the total hours spent on protected deep work. Professionals often report higher quality output and less emotional exhaustion when they enforce these simple but firm boundaries.

Resistance is common. Concerns such as "I'll miss something urgent" or "My boss expects instant replies" can be addressed by setting up status messages, using out-of-office responses during deep work blocks ("Currently engaged in focused work—please call my cell for urgent matters"), and gently educating others on how these practices ultimately improve response quality throughout the day.

Strategic "No" Framework

The ability to decline requests directly supports emotional and commitment boundaries. Framing each "no" as a tool for professional clarity—not avoidance or inflexibility—transforms refusal into an act of prioritization. Different situations require different scripts and follow-ups:

Scenario	Initial Response	If Pushed	Alternative Suggestion	Phrasing Style
Extra Work Request	"My current commitments mean I can't take this on right now."	"Given capacity, another deadline would affect quality."	"Could we schedule this for next month or delegate?"	Direct, firm
Meeting Invitation	"I'm unable to attend at that time. Can I review notes afterward?"	"If vital, happy to meet for 15 minutes only."	"Would an async update suffice?"	Collaborative, flexible
Unrealistic Deadline	"With current projects, I'd need more time to meet that deadline and maintain quality."	"My schedule won't allow for a rush without risking errors."	"Can I deliver a draft on Friday and final version Monday?"	Honest, solution-driven
After-Hours Contact	"I check messages during work hours; I'll respond in the morning."	"As a habit, I disconnect after hours to recharge."	"If this is urgent, please call directly or mark the email 'Urgent'."	Respectful, clear
Scope Creep	"That change isn't within project scope, but I can discuss adding it to our next phase."	"Let's revisit project objectives before expanding."	"Could we prioritize key changes first and revisit others next round?"	Boundaried, professional

In a corporate setting, an analyst may receive an after-hours email requesting a surprise weekend report. The analyst replies, "Thank you for flagging this. I check messages during office hours, so I will be able to review it on Monday." If urgent work is demanded, they follow up with, "I disconnect after hours to maintain focus. If this is a true emergency, please call me directly." In client services, a project lead is pressed on deadline changes; they respond, "Given our current priorities, a Friday draft and a Monday final delivery will maintain our quality standards."

Implementation steps begin with setting template responses in email tools and practicing their use in lower-stakes scenarios. Professionals can also rehearse boundary statements out loud—each repetition builds confidence and internalizes the strategy. Following up, especially if pressure is applied, should never waver from the main message: respect for time leads to better results.

Metrics for this approach include the frequency of unnecessary meetings declined, urgent work successfully deferred, and time spent on misaligned extras reduced. In most environments—remote, managerial, or client-facing—these skills create less burnout and higher job satisfaction.

Building strong digital and communication boundaries does not mean being less available; it means being fully present and resourceful when it matters most. These professional tactics set the stage for extending boundaries into personal domains, where digital detox and work-life separation become the next areas of focus.

Making Boundaries Visible, Sustainable, and Mappable

Being proactive about boundaries in professional settings means stating needs and expectations directly. For example, when managing workflow interruptions, a phrase like "I block focused work time between 2-4 PM daily to ensure project completion. Please hold non-urgent requests until after," signals your availability clearly. When colleagues expect instant replies, respond with "I reply to non-urgent emails within 24 hours so I can dedicate time for deep work." If a manager assigns an unexpected task, a boundary can sound like, "For optimal quality, I require two days' notice for new assignments." These statements eliminate ambiguity, reduce conflict, and keep workloads manageable.

Proactively using visual boundary cues supports these communications. Calendar blocking can show protected work time. Using tools like Google Calendar, professionals can label blocks as "Focus – Unavailable" so others see this reserved time. An office door with a "Do Not Disturb: Focused Work" sign helps curb interruptions in shared environments. Digitally, status indicators such as "Away" or "In Deep Work Mode" on collaboration platforms send real-time signals about availability. Time-blocking templates help divide days into segments for email management, meetings, and personal projects, making priorities visible to both you and your team.

Transforming boundaries from apologetic requests to confident policy statements requires conscious language shifts. Consider this evolution:

Apologetic Request	Confident Policy Statement
"I'm sorry, but I can't take on more projects now."	"My project capacity is currently full through Q3."
"I hope it's okay, but I need to leave at 5 today."	"I end all work commitments at 5 PM to honor my schedule."
"Sorry for the delay. I needed some time to reset."	"For quality output, I schedule breaks between intensive tasks."

Start by identifying your standards, then practice stating them firmly, without over-explaining or apologizing. This models self-respect and teaches colleagues to honor your limits.

The Boundary Mapping Exercise provides a framework for developing actionable boundaries:

Boundary Mapping Exercise

Exercise Purpose: Identify boundary needs and create clear, actionable solutions.

Implementation Steps:

List areas that cause stress or overwhelm.

Name the specific boundary violation present.

Write out your ideal boundary in clear, concise terms; for example: "I need all meeting requests to come with at least 24 hours' notice."

Identify tools (calendar blocks, status indicators) to support the boundary.

Communicate the boundary to relevant parties.

Success Metrics:

A noticeable decrease in interruptions or feelings of overwhelm.

Consistency in following the boundary over one workweek.

Positive feedback from colleagues regarding clarity.

Follow-up Actions:

Review and adjust boundaries weekly.

Seek feedback from trusted colleagues.

Adjust language or tools as situations change.

For hands-on practice, begin by documenting three overwhelming situations from the past week. For each situation, analyze which boundary was crossed. Define the ideal outcome for the next time this situation arises. Draft a boundary statement. For instance, if late meetings cut into personal time, a possible boundary could be, "I need all meetings to end by 5 PM." Practice implementing one boundary statement daily. This exercise builds confidence and consistency.

The Focus Protection Plan template cements boundaries:

Focus Protection Plan

Area	Example
Priority Time Blocks	9–11 AM, 2–4 PM: Deep Work (no meetings)
Communication Protocols	Reply to emails 11:30 AM/3:30 PM; IM for urgent only
Digital Boundaries	No notifications during focus blocks
Meeting Guidelines	Accept only meetings with agendas; none after 4 PM
Personal Time Protection	Lunch break 12–1 PM; phone off after 6 PM

Scripts for common scenarios make boundary-setting easier:

Situation: Last-minute meeting request.

Boundary Statement: "I require at least 24 hours' notice for meetings."

Alternatives: "Is this urgent? If so, we can touch base over chat."

Follow-up: After the meeting, remind the team of the preferred schedule.

Situation: A colleague sends chat messages during focus time.

Boundary Statement: "I'm in focused work time until 4 PM. Can we connect afterward?"

Alternatives: "Email me the details; I'll review them at 4 PM."

Follow-up: Reinforce the boundary if the pattern repeats.

Situation: A manager assigns extra work.

Boundary Statement: "My workload is full this week. Can we discuss priorities or a new timeline?"

Alternatives: "I'm open to shifting deadlines on lower-priority items."

Follow-up: Summarize agreements in writing for clarity.

The "bonus challenge" is to practice setting boundaries gracefully in real time. Try kind but firm responses like, "Thanks for thinking of me, but I can't take that on right now," or "No, I'm unavailable at that time, but I appreciate the invitation." This style maintains professionalism, demonstrates self-respect, and encourages mutual respect. Every exercise and tool in this section supports sustainable, actionable boundaries—essential skills for professionals balancing demanding roles and complex work environments.

Bringing It All Together

Now that we understand the critical role boundaries play in managing input overload and preserving well-being, busy professionals can intentionally design and enforce these limits to protect their time, focus, and emotional energy. By applying strategic approaches—such as setting clear time blocks, controlling information flow, and asserting emotional limits—individuals not only prevent burnout but also enhance productivity and job satisfaction. With consistent practice and visible communication of boundaries, professionals create sustainable work habits that support both personal health and career success. Embracing these boundary-setting skills positions busy men and women to thrive amid demanding environments while maintaining balance in their lives.

Chapter 6: Self-Compassion – Embracing Imperfection

Every professional has faced the relentless inner voice that demands more—more effort, more precision, more control. It whispers fears about mistakes and imperfections, urging you to push harder and never show vulnerability. This constant self-criticism often feels like motivation, but it quietly drains energy, fosters anxiety, and deepens feelings of failure. Many find themselves caught in cycles of overthinking, replaying errors, or drowning in doubts despite their achievements and capabilities.

This chapter examines the hidden impact of harsh self-judgment in professional life and introduces a different way of relating to yourself—a way rooted not in blame but in understanding and kindness. By exploring how to recognize and transform your inner dialogue, you will learn practical tools for embracing imperfection without losing your drive. The focus will be on building self-compassion skills that help reduce burnout, foster resilience, and create space for genuine growth amid the pressures and challenges of the workplace.

Understanding Self-Criticism and Practicing Real-Life Self-Compassion

The belief that tough self-criticism drives higher performance is deeply ingrained in professional culture. Many professionals assume that the voice urging them to "push harder" and "do better" is essential for success. However, research reveals the opposite: habitual self-criticism decreases productivity, increases burnout, and weakens resilience. Rather than acting as a motivator, self-criticism undermines the confidence and well-being needed to succeed at work. Studies document that individuals who rely on self-criticism experience more intense feelings of shame, anxiety, and emotional exhaustion, making it harder to bounce back from setbacks or maintain consistent performance.

Workplace pressure can create a mindset where mistakes seem catastrophic and any imperfection feels unacceptable. This reaction is closely linked to emotional perfectionism, which manifests as an internal fear of showing any negative emotion or vulnerability. Emotional perfectionism isn't about keeping your desk tidy; it's about expecting flawless emotional responses—never feeling anxious, never making mistakes, and always staying in control. In professional settings, this pushes people to hide their stress or overprepare for fear of disappointment. They may replay negative feedback in their heads, worry endlessly about minor errors in reports, or dwell on how a meeting could have gone better. This cycle of overthinking consumes energy and distracts from meaningful work. The pressure to "get it right" emotionally creates a breeding ground for burnout, while self-compassion offers a healthier alternative.

Self-compassion consists of three practical elements that can be immediately applied in the workplace. The first component is mindfulness. In a professional context, mindfulness means recognizing stress as it arises—such as during an impending project deadline—without trying to ignore or suppress it. For example, an employee racing to finish a report may notice rising tension and acknowledge, "This situation is stressful, but that's a normal reaction." Mindfulness keeps you present and curious about your emotions rather than swept away by them.

The second element, common humanity, involves understanding that setbacks are a universal part of the professional experience. It's easy to think you're the only one struggling when you miss a deadline or receive negative feedback. However, common humanity means remembering that every coworker, even those who seem at ease, faces challenges. Leaders who openly discuss their own learning moments create psychologically safe workplaces, encouraging others to ask for help or admit when they don't have all the answers. Knowing that struggle is normal diffuses shame and makes asking for support less intimidating.

The third component, self-kindness, involves treating yourself with the same support and patience you would offer a colleague. This might mean allowing yourself a five-minute break after an intense meeting or reassuring yourself after a presentation didn't go as planned. Self-kindness can sound like, "Everyone makes mistakes during presentations—this doesn't define my capabilities." When professionals respond to mistakes with encouragement instead of criticism, they feel safer to try new ideas, reducing the paralysis that comes from the fear of failure.

Misunderstandings about self-compassion are common in high-pressure environments. Many professionals fear that being kind to themselves will morph into self-pity or that they will start making excuses for poor performance. In reality, self-compassion does not mean indulging in self-pity or shifting responsibility onto others. Rather, it's an active process of caring for yourself while remaining accountable. When a professional misses a deadline, self-compassion involves acknowledging the disappointment, reflecting on what contributed to the delay, and planning a better approach for next time. This contrasts sharply with self-criticism, which might spiral into rumination, guilt, or avoidance—none of which promote learning or growth.

Self-compassion is also distinct from complacency. Instead of letting professionals "off the hook," research emphasizes that self-compassionate individuals are more likely to take responsibility, learn from their errors, and persist after failure. For example, when someone receives critical feedback on a project, self-criticism might prompt them to avoid future challenges out of fear. In contrast, self-compassion encourages reviewing the feedback objectively, making adjustments, and moving forward with less fear and more resilience.

In practical terms, many professionals respond to mistakes by replaying errors in their minds, trying to outwork their feelings of inadequacy, or simply shutting down. These instinctive reactions only entrench self-doubt and reduce motivation. By observing these patterns, it becomes possible to shift toward a compassionate internal dialogue—one that supports growth, reduces overthinking, and sustains well-being through professional ups and downs.

Changing Your Inner Dialogue: Methods and Reframe Practice

The pressure-packed environment of professional life places the inner critic in a prime position. Minor setbacks—such as slipping up in front of colleagues, missing a deadline, or sending an email without double-checking—inevitably activate self-critical thoughts. Distinguishing these moments is the first step in gaining control over the dialogue. Catching these triggers in real time often takes only a second of awareness, but this pause makes change possible. For instance, notice when you flinch after realizing you forgot to follow up with a client or when your heart sinks because you stumbled during a pitch. Identifying these triggers makes it easier to pinpoint when the inner critic is about to take over.

The 2-Minute Reframe Practice offers a swift, actionable approach to disrupting this negative pattern. Busy schedules leave little room for lengthy meditations, but this routine fits even into a packed calendar. Begin by selecting the trigger—perhaps you missed a project deadline and immediately think, "I always let the team down. I'm so disorganized." Recognize this harsh mental reprimand as your cue. Start the reframe by taking a slow, deliberate breath. Ask yourself if the thought is based on facts or if it's loaded with harsh assumptions. Challenge the statement directly: Is "always" even true? Recall completed projects, achievements, and past instances when you delivered successfully. Now, actively replace the critic's phrase with a supportive response. For example, change "I always let the team down" to "This was a tough week, and I missed the deadline, but I've handled high-pressure projects before. I can review the problem and improve my system".

For a step-by-step guide, keep these concrete actions on hand:

2-Minute Reframe Practice

Notice the Trigger

Pause when you detect a spike of self-blame after a work slip, such as faltering during a meeting.

Name the Critical Thought

Mentally capture the exact words. A common phrase is: "I completely messed up that explanation. Everyone thinks I'm incompetent."

Challenge and Investigate

Ask: Would I speak this way to a respected colleague or friend struggling with the same mistake? Usually, the answer is no.

Reframe with Compassion

Transform the criticism. Change "I completely messed up that explanation. Everyone thinks I'm incompetent" to "That answer could've been clearer, but mistakes are normal. I care about doing well, and this is an opportunity to clarify next time".

Set a timer if needed—two minutes is enough to keep the process both focused and manageable. Mark specific moments in your workday where self-critical spirals tend to appear: right after sending a rushed email, while commuting after a demanding meeting, or even in between tasks during a coffee break. By anchoring the reframe practice to these micro-moments, it slides seamlessly into even the most hectic routine.

For implementation in real-life scenarios, refer to this table of common workplace triggers and fast reframes:

Trigger	Critical Thought	Reframed Statement
Missing a deadline	"I'm hopeless at managing my time."	"Deadlines are stressful; I can identify what didn't work and adjust."
Forgetting to follow up with a client	"They'll think I'm careless and unreliable."	"Everyone overlooks things; I can apologize and make it right."
Making a mistake in a presentation	"I always mess up under pressure."	"That mistake was frustrating, but I kept going. I can learn from this."

| Stumbling during a meeting | "No one will take me seriously now." | "Presenting is challenging; I showed up and can prepare differently." |

Track progress by noting shifts in emotional tone after the practice. Even slight relief or a sense of perspective signals positive change—this is your progress marker. If the reframed statement feels awkward, that's normal. Over time, the new responses will begin to sound more authentic than the critic's harsh words.

The reframing process aligns with the pillars of self-compassion. Mindfulness appears in the very act of catching and objectively viewing the critical thought. Common humanity enters when you remember that mistakes are not signs of personal failure but part of the shared human experience that professionals navigate daily. Self-kindness takes shape in the transformed language—a gesture of patience and understanding toward yourself rather than condemnation.

By consistently practicing this reframing, the loop of harsh self-talk weakens. The voice that once sabotaged performance transforms into a quieter companion, offering constructive support instead of biting critique. Incremental improvements will begin to loosen the rigid hold of perfectionistic tendencies, making space for genuine resilience and growth.

Detoxing Perfectionism and Building Lasting Compassion Habits

Busy professionals often become entangled in perfectionist traps. One of the most common traps is setting standards so high that they become unachievable, such as reworking a project report repeatedly, convinced it will never be "good enough." Another trap is obsessing over minor details, like spending hours tweaking a slide font rather than preparing the content for a client presentation. There is also the trap of perpetual dissatisfaction, where even after exceeding expectations, the achievement feels empty. Project submissions are postponed indefinitely in the belief that one more revision will finally make the work flawless. Professionals may spend late nights redoing tasks that have already been completed, fearing that a missed detail will reflect poorly on them. These behaviors stem from thoughts like "I should never make mistakes" or "If I'm not exceptional, I'm nothing special".

The "Perfectionism Release Protocol" is designed to help break these ingrained patterns through identification, response, and practical change.

The Perfectionism Release Protocol

Behavior Identification

Compulsively double-checking or redoing work unnecessarily

Reluctance to delegate, convinced that only personal effort ensures quality

Delaying project submissions to perfect every detail

Downplaying achievements or dismissing praise

Experiencing anxiety or guilt after making small mistakes

Alternative Response

Accept "good enough" for non-critical tasks; define clear stopping points for edits

Delegate with specific instructions, trusting colleagues to deliver

Submit work by a firm deadline, resisting last-minute changes unless they are crucial

Practice accepting compliments with a simple "thank you"

Treat mistakes as learning moments without connecting them to self-worth

Implementation Strategy

Draft a checklist of daily perfectionist tendencies and post it visibly

Choose one behavior per week to consciously adjust, such as setting a timer for review periods to prevent over-editing

Partner with a colleague as an accountability buddy and communicate progress each Friday

Use reminders to accept praise or to pause and reflect before making "just one more" revision

Admit to a team member when a task is submitted as "good enough" rather than "perfect," and note the result

Progress Tracking Method

At the end of the workday, log which perfectionist behaviors were noticed and which alternative responses were practiced

Note small wins: delivering a report on time, delegating a task, or accepting positive feedback

Track feelings of anxiety or relief and look for patterns of improvement each week

The Kindness Audit

This exercise involves recording instances of harsh self-talk—the internal voice that calls a delayed email response "unprofessional" or magnifies a typo in a presentation as a "total failure".

Keep a notepad or phone app handy throughout the day

When noticing negative self-talk, jot down the situation and the harsh thought—for example, "After forgetting a meeting, I thought: 'I'm so disorganized—my boss will be disappointed'"

Next to each entry, write a compassionate alternative: "Everyone misses a meeting sometimes. I can apologize and send the notes"

Review the log at the end of the week to identify recurring triggers and note any progress in catching or rephrasing harsh thoughts.

Accountability Paired With Self-Compassion

Professionals can maintain standards without sliding into self-attack. When missing a presentation deadline, self-critical thinking might say, "I've let everyone down," but a supportive dialogue reframes this as, "The project ran over because I wanted it to be thorough. I'll communicate openly, adjust my workflow, and ask for help next time." If a mistake occurs in a client meeting, rather than thinking, "I always mess up," try saying, "I made an error, but I handled the follow-up professionally. I'll use this to better prepare in the future". Critical feedback from a supervisor may provoke thoughts of inadequacy, but shifting to, "This feedback is meant to help me grow. I'm allowed to be learning," fosters resilience. After missing sales targets, replace "I'm failing at my job" with "Everyone faces setbacks. What can I do differently, and how can I support myself through this process?"

Micro-Wins: Building a Daily Celebration Ritual

Perfectionism blocks the recognition of progress. Identifying micro-wins means looking for small, daily accomplishments—a well-facilitated team huddle, a positive client email, or finishing a challenging task. Each evening, pause to acknowledge these wins: write them down, share them with a colleague, or give yourself five minutes of guilt-free relaxation. These daily celebrations build momentum and serve as living evidence against the myth that only perfect outcomes are worthwhile.

Transforming the inner dialogue from harsh criticism to supportive encouragement rewrites professional habits while nurturing resilience and well-being. By combining self-accountability with compassion, professionals can maintain high standards, but with flexibility, kindness, and a genuine celebration of progress over perfection.

Bringing It All Together

Now that we understand the damaging effects of harsh self-criticism and the powerful role of self-compassion, busy professionals are equipped to shift their inner dialogue toward support and growth. Embracing mindfulness, common humanity, and self-kindness allows us to break free from overthinking and perfectionist traps that drain energy and undermine confidence. By practicing practical strategies like reframing critical thoughts and celebrating small wins, we create space for resilience, learning, and sustained well-being amid work pressures. Moving forward, integrating these compassionate habits into daily routines empowers professionals not only to meet high standards but also to do so with greater clarity, balance, and lasting fulfillment.

Chapter 7: Integration – Creating Sustainable Habits

"Have you ever felt overburdened by stress, your mind cluttered with what feels like endless tasks and responsibilities that never seem to end? Many professionals struggle to maintain a sense of calm amidst their hectic schedules, often finding themselves slipping back into old habits despite their best efforts. The pursuit of clarity and tranquility can appear daunting when life's demands scream for immediate attention.

In the following chapter, we will delve into the strategies necessary for transforming insights into habits and building a daily rhythm that fosters enduring clarity and calm. We'll focus on realistic habits that are not time-consuming but yield significant, lasting impacts. By understanding how to maintain progress and build sustainable practices, you can create a balanced, focused approach to handling daily challenges effectively."

Building Consistent Habits

To create sustainable habits, busy professionals must prioritize realistic consistency that supports clarity and calm. The transition from insight to habit is crucial; the key lies in overcoming "reset relapse," a phenomenon where old habits easily resurface. Incorporating James Clear's habit model—consisting of a Reminder (cue), Routine (behavior), and Reward (internal or external payoff)—provides a practical framework for habit formation.

Begin by recognizing the Reminder. For many, overthinking becomes the cue. The mental noise that spirals from task to task without resolution demands attention. In these moments, the cue isn't just stress but an awareness of the need for internal stillness. One approach is to pause and acknowledge these thoughts, labeling them as signals rather than sources of frustration.

Next, establish the Routine, which is the actionable behavior to redirect your energy. Grounding practices are vital here. Consider the simple yet effective method of deep breathing. When racing thoughts emerge, consciously engage in a deep breathing exercise. Inhale slowly for four counts, hold for four counts, and exhale for four counts. Repeat this cycle. This creates a break in the overwhelming stream and provides a physical anchor in the present moment.

The Reward follows as the internal payoff. As you practice deep breathing, notice the growing calmness and clarity. Decision-making becomes simpler, shedding the fog of confusion. This moment of peace serves as a natural reward, reinforcing the behavior. Each time this process is repeated, the habit strengthens, making overthinking less and less dominant in your routine.

Implementing structured routines such as a morning check-in, a midday clarity scan, and an evening wind-down enhances the habit cycle. Start the day with a morning check-in. Ask yourself, "What matters today?" Focus on forthcoming events or tasks that align with long-term goals. Document these priorities in a planner or digital tool. Knowing your focus for the day provides a clear path forward, minimizing distractions.

During the midday clarity scan, assess your focus and energy. At this point, the question to ask is, "Am I focused on what I can control?" Acknowledge areas where energy might be needlessly spent on uncontrollable factors. Redirect your effort toward tasks within your influence. This mindfulness practice reduces stress and enhances productivity while simultaneously altering unproductive midday routines.

For the evening wind-down, guide your thoughts with, "What can I release for the night?" Compile a list of incomplete tasks and consciously decide which can wait. Reflect on the successes of the day and areas for growth. By releasing concerns that linger into the night, mental clutter decreases, improving sleep and setting a positive trajectory for the next day. Crafting a bedtime routine tailored to relaxation—such as hot tea, reading, or gentle stretching—ensures a restful transition.

Let's consider a scenario: a reader notices frantic mental chatter as the cue. In response, they sit for a deep breathing exercise, feeling their pulse slow with each cycle. As calm spreads, the clutter reassembles into clarity. The reward is a newfound peace and an actionable step forward. These small, deliberate practices multiply their impact over time, transforming daily experiences. These methods cement resilience, making obstacles feel conquerable.

For consistent integration, avoid redundancy by preserving uniqueness in each routine's impact. Each practice must offer a fresh angle, continually improving mental stamina. These routines, once ingrained, shape identity, leveraging habits to navigate complexity with confidence.

Incorporating these principles into your daily life demands commitment but pays off with a sustainable sense of peace and effectiveness. Professionals often face an onslaught of demands vying for attention. Structured routines offer stability, becoming pillars around which chaos is reordered. The confidence derived from achieving small victories accumulates, empowering you to tackle larger challenges.

In the subsequent section, explore how to select your top three go-to tools on high-stress days. Crafting a "reset menu" empowers customization, giving you a curated set of strategies to draw from when needed most. As part of weekly reflections, assessing progress and making necessary adjustments ensures habits remain dynamic and applicable.

This integration of habits fosters long-term success. They are not an abrupt overhaul but incremental shifts that produce profound results. Ensuring each practice remains manageable yet meaningful is paramount. The routines become intuitive, requiring less conscious effort, akin to muscle memory for the mind.

Integrate these strategies seamlessly, adapting them to fit individual lifestyles. Each professional's day is unique; tailoring routines ensures they remain relevant and effective. Gradually, these routines evolve, guiding decision-making and stress management. Shift the focus from aspiration to action, transforming insight into impact.

By embedding these principles into your daily rhythm, embrace a proactive approach to stress and productivity. Consistency yields dividends, both in mental clarity and professional achievement. Overcoming reset relapse isn't a battle of willpower but a symphony of small habits harmonizing for sustained success.

Utilizing Your Toolkit

Integrating awareness and mindfulness into daily routines can transform moments of clarity into sustainable habits. Consistency, a cornerstone for forming lasting habits, thrives on simplicity—making it imperative to allocate just a few minutes each day. As busy professionals, you need practical methods to fit mindfulness into already packed schedules. Let's explore this by revisiting the framework of reminders, routines, and rewards to reinforce new behaviors.

To begin, let's identify personalized strategies for managing stress effectively. Recognizing that what works for one person might not work for another is crucial in tailoring effective stress-management tools. Start by identifying your top go-to strategies, such as engaging in mind dumps or practicing mindful breathing. Mind dumps involve writing down all current thoughts and worries to clear mental clutter, offering immediate relief from overwhelming mental noise. Likewise, mindful breathing can instantly calm the mind. By personalizing these techniques, you enhance their effectiveness and increase the likelihood of adoption.

Create a "reset menu" for those high-stress days when life feels particularly overwhelming. This menu should be as visible as possible—think sticky notes on your computer, phone alarms, or calendar nudges serving as constant reminders. Design it by listing your most common high-stress scenarios and selecting tools that cater to each one. For instance, if overthinking often disrupts your workday, the act of taking a few mindful breaths can swiftly redirect your focus and return you to a calmer, more centered state. By anticipating these scenarios and preparing responses, you will have a tangible, practical plan for when stress strikes.

Diving into the process, start by selecting your top three go-to tools. First, identify moments when mental noise crescendos. Next, implement grounding practices like a two-minute body scan or a quick walk outside. Observe the clarity and calm that follow these interventions. Grounding practices allow you to connect with the present, dialing back stress and promoting mental space. The effectiveness lies not just in the practice itself, but in the act of choosing to pause and reorient—demonstrating discipline and commitment to your well-being.

With your reset menu, you can strategically prepare for situations that demand extra resilience. List stress-heavy scenarios, such as back-to-back meetings or pressing deadlines. For each scenario, select an appropriate tool that can be deployed in minutes and suits your needs. For instance, a two-minute S.T.O.P. practice can provide a mental pause, while observing a leaf outdoors briefly during lunch can recenter your attention. By organizing these tools visibly, they become embedded in your environment, making their use habitual rather than reactive.

To further illustrate, picture a typical stressful catalyst at work—perhaps an unexpected, challenging email. By consciously deciding to follow it with a brief breathing exercise, you set a precedent. Start with three deep breaths, allowing each inhale and exhale to fill and empty your lungs completely. This turns a common stressor into an opportunity for regaining control, effectively minimizing its power over your day. This practice, drawn from the three-minute breathing space, aligns your physical response with mental clarity.

Another practical exercise involves practicing mindfulness with a leaf or performing a short mindful eating session. Selecting an object like a leaf or a mini snack allows you to focus intently on its texture, color, and smell for a few minutes. Such exercises emphasize fully immersive experiences, blocking external noise and honing attention on current sensations. The act of being fully present during these times offers immediate stress reduction and fosters a habit of mindfulness even during mundane moments.

Embedding these exercises into daily life ensures that they aren't just temporary fixes but sustainable habits. The example of taking a mindful pause—say, standing for a minute to observe a tree outside in the midst of a hectic schedule—can transform into a ritualistic break. Over time, this practice cultivates a naturally occurring habit where you instinctively turn to these tools when stress emerges, ultimately lowering overall stress levels and reinforcing emotional resilience.

Keep in mind that the nature of sustainable habits lies in their adaptability. As life evolves and presents new challenges, so must your strategies adapt. Being flexible and open to modifying your reset menu keeps your practices relevant and responsive to current needs. Perhaps a new tool, such as a mindfulness bell—where you listen to the sound fade into silence—will be more effective some weeks than others. Embracing this fluid approach ensures that practices remain fresh and engaging rather than stale obligations.

In conclusion, the key to creating sustainable habits for clarity and calm lies in the thoughtful integration of awareness into daily life. By recognizing personal stress triggers and equipping yourself with practical tools, you create a proactive rather than reactive mindfulness practice. Such consistency cultivates not just momentary calm but long-term emotional fortitude, enhancing clarity in day-to-day decisions. Remember, the true value of these exercises emerges over time. Commit to these daily rituals, and witness the benefits unfold in your personal and professional life.

Overcoming Challenges and Resources

In the rush of daily life, constructing sustainable habits becomes essential for preserving personal growth. The challenge is not merely to incorporate these habits but to reshape them as pillars for an enduring and balanced life. As readers journey through this chapter, the focus shifts to embedding learned insights into manageable routines, allowing for minimal disruption and maximum impact.

Begin by recalling the strategies for reframing expectations you've encountered. Imagine a day when things haven't gone as planned; this is an opportunity to reset. Invoke the "48-hour rule" as a practical approach to ensure you resume your routine swiftly. By restarting any delayed habits within two days of disruption, the aspects of consistency and adaptability merge, with self-compassion acting as the cornerstone. This approach redefines setbacks as opportunities rather than failures.

Self-compassion weaves its way into maintaining these habits by encouraging gentleness with oneself, especially during challenging times. Remind yourself of the "Weekly Reset Planner," a tool designed to enhance reflection and planning skills. Dedicate 15 minutes each week to note achievements, recognize any deviations, and adjust upcoming tasks accordingly. This exercise promotes a cycle of acknowledgment and growth, preventing burnout and encouraging a growth mindset.

When it comes to goal-setting, simplifying the task can mitigate feelings of overwhelm. Start with the simplest version of a task and decide what would happen if you allowed B or even B-minus work. Use questions like, "What's a small step I can take today?" It's about focusing on progress over perfection, honoring your current capability, and allowing room for growth as clarity returns.

Consider incorporating routine check-ins with yourself throughout the day. Using a straightforward system, such as rating your energy levels on a scale from 1 to 10, provides quick insights into your mental and physical state. When you detect a significant dip, view it as a signal to pause and recalibrate. Frequent mini-resets, such as taking deep breaths between tasks, offer the rejuvenation needed to continue effectively.

Creating a "Build-a-Habit Menu" can simplify decision-making. List habits tailored to fit your lifestyle and immediate needs. Whether integrating daily meditation for mental clarity or reserving time for hobbies, this menu serves as a personal resource for fostering well-being. For example, if you notice overthinking triggers, refer to your menu to select calming practices that have been effective previously.

Ground yourself with realistic and adaptable exercises. Through structured tasks, establish a rhythm that accommodates fluctuations in personal and professional domains. Use clear, direct language and avoid complex participle phrases to maintain clarity. Real-world examples embedded within your lifestyle should guide your method creation.

Picture your day starting with gratitude exercises. Just five minutes spent expressing thankfulness for simple pleasures, akin to savoring morning coffee or feeling fresh sheets, can shift the mood of your entire day. It's crucial to appreciate life's small joys, which act as a counterbalance to difficult times and reinforce emotional stability.

The value of relationships becomes evident through intentional and nourishing connections. Schedule regular interactions with loved ones to bolster emotional support and reduce the impacts of isolation. Whether through shared meals or brief conversations, these interactions are exchanges of energy and are vital for mental well-being.

When busy schedules threaten to overwhelm, prioritize your to-do list by focusing on meaningful tasks. Resist the urge to tackle quick items first; instead, channel your energy toward the projects of highest importance. Prioritizing in this manner not only enhances productivity but also aligns with a more fulfilled sense of accomplishment. Doing what truly matters guides the rhythm of your daily life.

In moments of strain and extensive responsibility, granting yourself permission to pause becomes an act of self-care. Evaluate instances where taking a deliberate break proved beneficial. These intervals can restore energy and perspective, illustrating how balanced pacing contributes more effectively to your objectives. Pause, breathe, reset—likewise assess how adjustments to routines can optimize your narrative of growth.

Returning to tools that guide success fosters a sustainable path forward. Your "Weekly Reset Planner," accompanied by the strategic methods within this chapter, fortifies your commitment to yourself. At the heart, self-compassion is integral, transforming your past encouragements into constants when faced with challenging days.

Remember that each step, while small, ties into a larger framework of ongoing progress. Moreover, simplicity crowns complexity in daily routines. By investing in structured yet adjustable daily habits, you create a space for new insights and broader expansion of what you currently hold. These systematic steps ensure that any chaos in life can be met with calm resilience and alignment with your innermost values.

Incorporate awareness and insight into your rhythm today, allowing them to evolve and shape tomorrow's forward momentum.

Bringing It All Together

In closing, as you embrace the journey of building sustainable habits into your daily life, remember that consistency is key, and even small, intentional actions can yield significant results. By integrating the principles outlined in this chapter, you have equipped yourself with practical tools to maintain clarity amid the chaos and cultivate calmness through mindful routines. As busy professionals, shifting from insight to impactful action allows you to transform stress into manageable moments, fostering a resilient mindset for any challenge. Moving forward, continue to prioritize realistic habits that fit seamlessly into your unique schedules, enabling you to navigate life's complexities with confidence and purpose. With commitment and adaptability, these practices will not only enhance your professional efficiency but also enrich your personal well-being, crafting a balanced life filled with clarity and achievement.

Bonus Section: Your Reset Toolkit & Ongoing Support

Amid the constant hustle and bustle of daily life, maintaining momentum after committing to a lifestyle change can often feel like an uphill battle. Imagine the scenario: you've just completed a week-long reset, full of enthusiasm and determination. The joy of achievement is palpable, but as each day unfolds, familiar patterns begin to creep back in. Work demands escalate, mental clutter accumulates, and before you know it, the progress made seems to slip through your fingers. This scenario resonates with countless busy professionals who strive for consistent growth but find themselves navigating a maze of challenges.

In this chapter, we delve into the essential toolkit designed to help maintain and enhance your progress following that initial transformational reset. With a focus on practical tools and ongoing support, you'll discover ways to seamlessly integrate strategies into your routine, enabling sustained growth amidst life's demands. Whether it's harnessing the power of mindfulness or setting meaningful boundaries, these approaches are tailored to fit into even the most hectic schedules. Join us as we explore these insightful methods aimed at fostering resilience and ensuring continuous personal and professional development.

Introduction to the Concept of Completing the 7-Day Reset

Congratulations on completing your 7-day reset! This isn't just an endpoint; it's a significant stepping stone toward more profound, ongoing self-improvement. To ensure sustained progress, you'll need quick-reference tools that seamlessly fit into your packed schedule. Think of this section as your personal toolkit for resilience, designed to help you navigate both professional and personal challenges with ease.

One indispensable tool is the Mind Dump Journal. The main goal here is to clear your mental clutter efficiently within five minutes. Simply grab a notebook or digital device and jot down everything that's occupying your mind—tasks, reminders, worries, and ideas. This helps cleanse the mental palette, leaving space for creativity and focus. Do this at the start or end of your day, and you'll notice a significant improvement in clarity and decision-making. This practice isn't just about organizing thoughts; it's also an effective way to manage acute stress by externalizing and confronting anxieties on paper rather than letting them simmer internally.

Consider incorporating the Daily Reset Menu into your routine. This consists of three core components that will ensure you maintain focus from dawn to dusk. Start with a Morning Check-In, where you identify your priorities and set a clear focus for your day. Ask yourself, "What matters today?" This helps ground your actions in what truly requires your attention and avoids unnecessary distractions.

The Midday Clarity Scan comes next. Take a brief moment to assess your progress around noon. Are you solving problems or merely spiraling in loops? This scan keeps your decisions aligned with your overarching goals, preventing burnout and misdirection. Concluding your day, the Evening Wind-Down is your time to release accumulated stressors. Ask yourself, "What can I release for the night?" Acknowledging the pressures and intentionally setting them aside prepares your mind and body for restorative sleep.

Our top techniques are also purpose-built for ongoing use and can be seamlessly integrated into your lifestyle. Consider the 3-2-1 Decision Method. It's a structured solution to avoid overthinking. Start by listing three tasks or decisions. For each, identify two viable options. For one minute per task, weigh the options, then make your decision. This method limits the time spent dwelling on decisions, enhancing productivity and reducing decision fatigue.

Boundaries are another vital area. Use Boundary Scripts to assertively define your limits. Direct examples may include: "I'm unable to take that on right now, but let's revisit it tomorrow," or "I need this time to focus on my priorities." Clarifying boundaries ensures you manage your time and energy wisely, preventing burnout and maintaining healthy relationships, whether at home or in the office.

Integrating these tools requires avoiding redundancy while focusing on the core benefits each offers. For example, each of the mentioned techniques aids in decision-making but in distinct ways—whether by organizing thoughts, reinforcing intention, or clarifying limits. They also adapt to various professional settings, from corporate roles requiring quick decision-making to creative jobs needing mental space for inspiration.

A curious mind might wonder—how deep can these tools truly take you? It's worth mentioning that suggested readings complement this toolkit. Delving into these can deepen your understanding and proficiency, enriching your practice without overshadowing the current practical exercises we've focused on here.

By embedding these methods into your daily habits, you'll not merely survive the workweek but thrive consistently. Let each exercise serve as a catalyst for lifelong sustainable success, turning ordinary days into productivity-rich, stress-minimized experiences. This toolkit is not a one-size-fits-all; it's versatile enough to meet your unique rhythm and demands, growing with you as your professional and personal life evolves.

Enhance your endeavors with these practical strategies, and invite reflection, refinement, and revitalization into your everyday life. As you continue evolving past your initial reset, these exercises will become second nature, providing ongoing support and fostering resilience. Now, you have the essentials to keep moving forward in a balanced, composed manner every single day.

Suggested Reading List and Maintaining Progress

The "Bonus Section: Your Reset Toolkit & Ongoing Support" builds upon earlier discussions by emphasizing the importance of continuous growth in personal development. You have already been introduced to core tools like the Daily Reset Menu, which laid the groundwork for this journey. Now, let's consider some essential readings. These resources dive deeper into self-compassion, habit formation, priority setting, and mindfulness, each offering specific strategies to help us thrive amidst daily demands. The journey we started does not conclude after the initial 7-day reset; instead, these readings serve as companions on your ongoing path to self-improvement.

Brené Brown's "The Gifts of Imperfection" makes a great starting point. Brown emphasizes self-compassion as a cornerstone of personal growth. She challenges the notion of perfectionism, encouraging us to embrace vulnerability as a strength rather than a weakness. In a bustling work environment, it is easy to get tangled up in trying to meet unrealistic standards. Brown provides a shift in perspective, advocating for authenticity and self-acceptance. Imagine a busy professional navigating an intense workweek. Instead of succumbing to a cycle of self-criticism when things go awry, they can channel Brown's insights, opting to view mistakes as opportunities to learn and grow. This mindset shift not only alleviates pressure but also enhances productivity and mental well-being.

Moving on to James Clear's "Atomic Habits," we explore the science of habit formation. Clear's approach is grounded in the idea that small, consistent changes lead to remarkable results. He introduces the concept of "atomic habits"—those tiny changes that compound over time. For busy professionals, developing good habits can be the difference between chaos and harmony in their daily lives. Imagine starting a morning routine, beginning with just five minutes of meditation. By incrementally building on small habits, you create sustainable and positive momentum. Clear's strategies empower us to design environments that naturally support beneficial behaviors, ultimately leading to significant lifestyle improvements.

Greg McKeown's "Essentialism" offers another powerful tool by focusing on the art of priority setting. In McKeown's view, being busy does not equate to being productive. Instead, he argues for discerning what is truly essential and eliminating the non-essential. For professionals, this means making deliberate choices about where to invest time and energy. Imagine a situation where work demands seem overwhelming. Applying McKeown's principles, you would pause to assess which tasks align with long-term goals, allowing you to cut through the noise and concentrate on high-impact activities. This not only boosts effectiveness but also fosters improved work-life balance, providing a clearer path to achieving both personal and professional aspirations.

Tara Brach's "Radical Acceptance" delves into emotional mindfulness, offering a strategy to embrace our full spectrum of emotions with compassion. She underscores the importance of acknowledging feelings rather than dismissing them. For many professionals, the constant pursuit of success can lead to emotional suppression. Brach encourages leaning into vulnerability, allowing us to experience emotions authentically. Picture a moment of stress, perhaps during a major project deadline. Instead of repressing anxiety, we can acknowledge it, channeling that energy into productive action. This approach nurtures resilience, allowing us to navigate challenges with greater grace and adaptability.

Together, these readings facilitate self-improvement, inspiring readers to actively engage in their personal development journey beyond an initial reset phase. The insights from these books align with ongoing support, encouraging professionals to incorporate lessons into their daily lives. Each fosters resilience, rendering us better equipped to handle the pressures of our environments. By adopting the principles offered in these resources, individuals can sustain the progress initiated during the reset and continue evolving with intention and purpose.

The significance of this reading list lies in the mindset shift it promotes. Brown, Clear, McKeown, and Brach do not just offer strategies; they provide frameworks for rethinking how we approach challenges. Their insights encourage a paradigm shift, vital for long-term success. Armed with these perspectives, we become proactive in shaping our lives, identifying what truly matters, and moving confidently toward our ambitions. For busy professionals, this invests power in flexibility, an essential trait in ever-changing environments.

As we wrap up this reading exploration, it is crucial to transition into the forthcoming content. Next, you will learn about community and accountability through participation in activities like the Reset Circle and Monthly Mini-Resets. Engaging with a supportive community enhances your ability to apply insights from these readings, grounding theory in practice. It is one thing to gain knowledge from a book; it is another to see how peers implement these ideas, experiencing their challenges and triumphs alongside them.

Joining the Reset Circle or participating in Monthly Mini-Resets further enriches your journey, drawing from shared experiences and collective wisdom. They offer platforms to test new strategies, seek feedback, and celebrate successes with like-minded individuals. In this way, engagement with these communities fosters accountability, ensuring you remain aligned with your goals. Such participation bridges the current discussion with the practical next steps, opening a gateway to sustained personal and professional growth.

Maintaining progress requires a commitment to lifelong learning and adaptation. By embracing the tools and insights offered by Brown, Clear, McKeown, and Brach, and engaging with community support systems, you set a strong foundation for continuous evolution, ensuring the journey not only persists but thrives. As we explore the upcoming sections, remember this: the path of development is ongoing, fueled by curiosity, resilience, and a desire to better both ourselves and the environments around us.

Staying Connected and Final Action Step

Imagine you're embarking on a continuous journey of self-improvement and growth. After the initial burst from a 7-day reset program, it's about maintaining momentum and infusing these positive changes into daily living. The ultimate goal is to create a toolkit filled with practical resources, emotional support, and a strong sense of community that keeps you connected with your progress and others.

Beginning with self-compassion and healthy boundaries, think about the insights gained from Brené Brown's teachings on imperfection and vulnerability. As we navigate the pressures of professional life, maintaining self-kindness allows us to acknowledge setbacks without judgment and move forward constructively. Following this mindset helps frame our goals and boundaries as acts of respect for our own time and energy.

Drawing from James Clear's "Atomic Habits," incorporate micro-actions into your routine. These small, intentional steps can bridge the daunting gap between intention and action. Rather than overhauling your entire routine or setting ambitious but unattainable goals, integrate actions like spending five minutes meditating or jotting down a few gratitude notes each evening. Research underscores the value of these brief practices for enhancing mood and focus. Consistently piecing together these micro-actions can transform them into powerful, sustainable habits over time.

Next, consider Greg McKeown's "Essentialism" as a guide to concentrating on tasks that truly matter. By evaluating responsibilities through a lens of essentialism, you can pursue impactful endeavors, thus freeing yourself from the noise of non-essential tasks. This doesn't just simplify decision-making; it removes distractions that can otherwise fragment your attention and heighten stress.

Mindfulness serves as a cornerstone for sustaining growth. Tara Brach's "Radical Acceptance" highlights the value of presence — accepting our experiences with compassion. For professionals, this means navigating work stress calmly, improving decision-making, and enhancing emotional intelligence. Studies show that mindfulness enhances resilience, empowering you to bounce back from setbacks with grace and clarity.

To anchor these principles into actionable steps, let's dive into some carefully designed exercises. "Join the Reset Circle" extends an invitation into an online community where participants share their pathways, challenges, and wins. Regular interaction in this space amplifies personal commitment. Experiencing growth alongside others fosters mutual encouragement and underscores that meaningful change doesn't happen in isolation.

Another practical strategy is "Subscribe for Monthly Mini-Resets." These monthly engagements are brief yet impactful, offering bite-sized prompts and resources to maintain motivation. They serve to refresh your commitment, preventing complacency. Clear steps for accessing these resources make them easy to incorporate into your packed schedule, thus ensuring consistency without feeling overburdened.

For those willing to explore further, "Want to Go Deeper?" encourages engaging with premium resources like workbooks or courses. These delve into topics more intricately and provide a scaffold for solidifying new habits. Such in-depth exploration supports a fuller understanding and implementation of strategies that underpin sustained personal development.

Reflective practices also play a key role. Crafting a "Reset Letter" is an exercise in self-accountability. Through reflective writing, consider your mindset shifts, memories worth preserving, and effective strategies you've discovered. These letters become personal artifacts — reminders of growth that can be revisited during challenging times, promoting self-awareness and recalibration.

Each of these exercises functions as a staircase, each step propelling you upwards towards a lifestyle where actions align with core values. The strategies move beyond theory, making them tangible and applicable to even the busiest individuals. The beauty lies in their adaptability; they respect your time, merging seamlessly into existing routines without causing overwhelm.

The challenge, of course, is consistency. Transformation thrives on continuous effort rather than sporadic bursts of change. Avoiding redundancy is essential. Instead, embrace clarity and try to ensure that each activity adds depth and direction to your journey without reverting to commonplace advice.

Reconsider the emphasis on mindfulness. Mindfulness isn't just a tool; it's a lens that reframes daily interactions, reshaping them into opportunities for growth. As studies show, even short bursts of mindfulness improve mood and focus, which, in turn, enhances overall well-being. Coupling mindfulness with other growth strategies can yield a rounded toolkit capable of addressing various facets of life, both personal and professional.

These practices signify moving beyond mere advice into action. They inspire adopting a mindset of continuous improvement and self-discovery. The enduring sentiment is progress, not perfection. In setting realistic, achievable milestones, professionals find not just one-time solutions but lasting improvements to their quality of life. Over time, this balanced approach can bring forth profound personal and professional transformation.

Bringing It All Together

As we close this chapter, you are now equipped with an essential toolkit designed to sustain and enhance your progress beyond the 7-day plan. Integrating tools like the Mind Dump Journal and Daily Reset Menu into your daily routine will significantly aid in freeing mental space, setting clear priorities, and managing stress effectively. The practices of boundary-setting and decision-making strategies, such as the 3-2-1 Decision Method, will further streamline your journey by promoting clarity and focus. Coupled with reading resources from Brené Brown, James Clear, Greg McKeown, and Tara Brach, you will gain valuable insights to foster self-compassion, habit formation, essentialism, and mindfulness. Now, armed with these powerful strategies, continue to evolve by applying them seamlessly in your personal and professional life, guiding you toward sustained success, balance, and fulfillment.

From the Author, Grant Merrill

If you've reached this page, I want to pause and say something simple but powerful: **well done.**

You didn't just start something—you stuck with it. Through busy days, off weeks, and all the mental clutter life throws your way, you keep returning. And that says more about your strength than any number, scale, or checklist ever could.

This plan wasn't created just from research or good intentions—it was born from real experience. I know what it's like to want change but feel stuck. To crave structure but feel overwhelmed. To get halfway through a plan and think, *"I'm not sure this is working."* But the truth is: it was. And it is.

The Overthinker's Rescue Plan was never about being perfect. It's about becoming consistent. It's about remembering that taking care of yourself doesn't have to mean pushing harder—it can mean pausing, checking in, and choosing progress over pressure.

If this book helped you realign your energy, rediscover your strength, or simply make wellness feel *doable* again, I'd be deeply grateful if you left a short, honest review on Amazon. Not just for me—but for the next woman who's deciding whether she's ready to commit to herself.

You can scroll down the book's Amazon page and click "Write a customer review." A few words about what worked for you could be exactly what she needs to say yes.

Thank you for trusting me to guide you through these 7-day plan. Whether this is the end of your first day—or the start of your next one—remember: *you already have what it takes. Now you have the rhythm to keep going.*

See you in the next book,
Grant Merrill

About the Author

Grant Merrill is the author of multiple wellness and lifestyle books designed to help everyday women build sustainable habits—one small, intentional step at a time. With a master's degree in management and a passion for personal development, Grant combines strategic thinking with empathetic coaching to make lasting change feel both achievable and empowering.

Rooted in the rhythms of seasonal living from his years in the Northeast, Grant's approach to wellness is refreshingly human-first: practical, gentle, and grounded in real life. His work focuses on helping beginners overcome overwhelm, guiding readers to reframe fitness, nourishment, and reflection as acts of self-respect—not self-punishment.

When he's not writing, Grant is coaching clients, diving into the latest research on habit psychology, or wandering a local farmers' market with a hot cup of coffee in hand.

www.ingramcontent.com/pod-product-compliance
Lightning Source LLC
Chambersburg PA
CBHW071314110426
42743CB00042B/1995